UNDERSTANDING THE PHYSIOLOGY OF THE ENDOCRINE SYSTEM

Authors:

Mark Aquino

Alada Johnson

Shittu Lorenzo

Publisher:

Elight Enterprise

Publication Date: July 2024

© 2024 by Elight Enterprise. All rights reserved.

Copyright Page

© 2024 by Elight Enterprise. All rights reserved.

No part of this book may be reproduced, stored in a retrieval system, or transmitted in any form or by any means, electronic, mechanical, photocopying, recording, or otherwise, without the prior written permission of the publisher.

Published by:

Elight Enterprise

123 Publishing Avenue

Oyo city, Ibadan

First Edition: June 2024

ISBN (Paperback): 9798329264050

ISBN (Hardcover): 9798329264357

The information contained in this book is provided for educational and informational purposes only and is not intended as medical advice. The author and publisher disclaim any liability arising directly or indirectly from the use of this book.

Cover design by Elight Enterprise

For more information about our publications, please visit our website at www.elightenterprise.com

Table of Content

UNDERSTANDING THE PHYSIOLOGY OF THE ENDOCRINE SYSTEM 1

   Authors: 1

      Mark Aquino 1

      Alada Johnson 1

      Shittu Lorenzo 1

   Publisher: 1

      Elight Enterprise 1

   Publication Date: July 2024 1

Table of Content 3

Dedication 18

Preface 19

Chapter 1 20

   1.1 Introduction to Endocrinology 20

   1.2 Hormones: Definition, Classification, and Functions 20

      Classification of Hormones: 21

      Functions of Hormones: 22

   1.3 Mechanisms of Hormone Action 23

      Cell Surface Receptors: 23

      Intracellular Receptors: 26

      Nuclear Receptors: 27

   1.4 Regulation of Hormone Secretion 28

      Hypothalamus-Pituitary Axis 28

      Regulation of Hormone Secretion: 29

      Releasing and Inhibiting Factors 29

      Negative Feedback 30

- Circadian Rhythms and Environmental Cues ... 31
- Stress Response ... 32
- 1.5 Feedback Mechanisms in the Endocrine System ... 33
  - Negative Feedback Mechanism: ... 34
  - Positive Feedback Mechanism: ... 35
- 1.6 Conclusion ... 36
- Case Studies ... 36
  - Case Study 1: Feedback Mechanisms in Hormonal Regulation ... 36
  - Case Study 2: Hormonal Regulation in Stress Response ... 37
- Practice Questions for Self-Assessment ... 39
  - Multiple Choice Questions ... 39
  - Short Answer Questions ... 40
  - True or False Questions ... 40
- Answers ... 40
  - Case Study 1 ... 40
  - Case Study 2 ... 41
  - Multiple Choice Questions ... 42
  - Short Answer Questions ... 42
  - True or False Questions ... 43
- Bibliography ... 43
- Chapter 2 ... 45
- 2.1 Overview of Hormonal Assays ... 45
  - Types of Hormonal Assays: ... 45
  - Advantages of Hormonal Assays: ... 46
  - Limitations and Challenges: ... 48
  - Future Directions in Hormonal Assays: ... 48
- 2.2 Immunoassay Techniques ... 49

- Enzyme-Linked Immunosorbent Assay (ELISA) 49
- Radioimmunoassay (RIA) 51
- Chemiluminescent Immunoassay (CLIA) 52
- 2.5 Mass Spectrometry 53
  - Principles of Mass Spectrometry: 54
  - Liquid Chromatography-Tandem Mass Spectrometry (LC-MS/MS): 54
  - Advantages of Mass Spectrometry in Hormonal Assays: 54
  - Challenges and Considerations: 54
- 2.6 Conclusion 55
- Case Studies 55
  - Case Study 1: Diagnosing Cushing's Syndrome 55
  - Case Study 2: Assessing Thyroid Function 56
- Practice Questions for Self-Assessment 57
  - Multiple Choice Questions 57
  - Short Answer Questions 58
  - True or False Questions 59
- Answers 59
  - Case Study 1 59
  - Case Study 2 60
  - Multiple Choice Questions 60
  - Short Answer Questions 60
  - True or False Questions 61
- Bibliography 61
- Chapter 3 63
- 3.1 Anatomy and Function of the Hypothalamus 63
  - Anatomy of the Hypothalamus 63
- 3.2 Hypothalamic Hormones and their Regulation 65

3.3 Anatomy and Connectivity of the Hypothalamo-Pituitary Axis: 67

3.4 Role of the Hypothalamus in Stress Response 69

    Activation of the HPA Axis: 69

    Stimulation of the Adrenal Cortex: 70

    Negative Feedback Regulation: 70

    Impact of Chronic Stress: 70

3.5 Conclusion 71

Case Studies 71

    Case Study 1: Hypothalamic Dysfunction and Pituitary Regulation 71

    Case Study 2: Hypothalamic-Pituitary-Adrenal Axis Dysfunction 72

Practice Questions for Self-Assessment 74

    Multiple Choice Questions 74

    Short Answer Questions 75

    True or False Questions 75

Answers 75

    Case Study 1 75

    Case Study 2 76

    Multiple Choice Questions 77

    Short Answer Questions 77

    True or False Questions 78

Bibliography 78

Chapter 4 79

4.1 Anatomy and Structure of Adenohypophysis: 79

    Anatomy: 79

    Cell Types: 80

4.2 Hormones Produced by Adenohypophysis: 80

    Growth Hormone (GH): 81

- Prolactin (PRL): 81
- Thyroid-Stimulating Hormone (TSH): 81
- Adrenocorticotropic Hormone (ACTH): 82
- Luteinizing Hormone (LH) and Follicle-Stimulating Hormone (FSH): 82

4.3 Regulation of Adenohypophyseal Hormones: 82
- Hypothalamic Control: 82
- Peripheral Regulation: 83
- Feedback Mechanisms: 83

4.4 Conclusion 83

Case Studies 84
- Case Study 1: Growth Hormone Dysregulation 84
- Case Study 2: Hypopituitarism 85

Practice Questions for Self-Assessment 86
- Multiple Choice Questions 86
- Short Answer Questions 87
- True or False Questions 88

Answers 88
- Case Study 1 88
- Case Study 2 89
- Multiple Choice Questions 89
- Short Answer Questions 90
- True or False Questions 90

Bibliography 91

Chapter Five 92

5.1 Anatomy and Structure of the Neurohypophyseal System: 92
- Location and Connections: 92
- Histological Composition: 92

- Nerve Fibers and Terminals: 92
- Vascular Supply: 93
- Relationship with Hypothalamic Nuclei: 93

5.2 Hormones Produced by Neurohypophysis: 93
- Oxytocin 93
- Vasopressin (Antidiuretic Hormone, ADH): 95

5.3 Regulation of Neurohypophyseal Hormone Secretion: 97
- Oxytocin Secretion Regulation: 98
- Vasopressin (Antidiuretic Hormone, ADH) Secretion Regulation: 99

5.4 Conclusion 100

Case Studies 101
- Case Study 1: Diabetes Insipidus 101
- Case Study 2: Syndrome of Inappropriate Antidiuretic Hormone Secretion (SIADH) 102

Practice Questions for Self-Assessment 103
- Multiple Choice Questions 103
- Short Answer Questions 104
- True or False Questions 104

Answers 105
- Case Study 1 105
- Case Study 2 105
- Multiple Choice Questions 106
- Short Answer Questions 106
- True or False Questions 107

Bibliography 107

Chapter 6 109

6.1 Growth Hormone: Structure and Synthesis 109
- Structure of Growth Hormone: 109

Synthesis of Growth Hormone: 110

6.2 Mechanisms of Action of Growth Hormone: 112

    Direct Effects of Growth Hormone: 112

    Integration of Direct and Indirect Effects: 113

6.3 Regulation of Growth Hormone Secretion 113

    Neural Regulation: 113

    Hormonal Regulation: 114

    Metabolic Regulation: 114

    6.4 Growth Factors 115

    Insulin-like Growth Factors (IGFs): 115

    Epidermal Growth Factors (EGFs): 117

    Fibroblast Growth Factors (FGFs): 118

    Transforming Growth Factor-Beta (TGF-β): 119

    Other Growth Factors: 120

Case Study 123

    Case Study 1: Growth Hormone Deficiency in a Child 123

    Case Study 2: Acromegaly in an Adult 125

Practice Questions for Self-Assessment 126

    Multiple Choice Questions 126

    Short Answer Questions 127

    True or False Questions 128

Answers 128

    Case Study 1 128

    Case Study 2 129

    Multiple Choice Questions 129

    Short Answer Questions 130

    True or False Questions 130

- Bibliography 131
- Chapter 7 132
  - Introduction: 132
  - 7.1 Anatomy and Histology of Thyroid Gland: 132
    - Anatomy of the Thyroid Gland: 132
    - Histology of the Thyroid Gland: 133
  - 7.2 Thyroid Hormones: Synthesis and Secretion 135
  - 7.3. Regulation of Thyroid Hormone Secretion: 136
  - 7.4 Thyroid Hormone Functions and Metabolic Effects: 137
  - 7.5 Conclusion 139
  - Case Studies 140
    - Case Study 1: Hyperthyroidism 140
    - Case Study 2: Hypothyroidism 141
  - Practice Questions for Self-Assessment 143
    - Multiple Choice Questions 143
    - Short Answer Questions 144
    - True or False Questions 144
  - Answers 145
    - Case Study 1 145
    - Case Study 2 145
    - Multiple Choice Questions 146
    - Short Answer Questions 146
    - True or False Questions 147
  - Bibliography 147
- Chapter Eight 150
  - 8.1 Anatomy and Zones of Adrenal Cortex: 150
    - 1. Zona Glomerulosa: 150

- 2. Zona Fasciculata: 150
- 3. Zona Reticularis: 151

8.2 Adrenal Steroid Hormones: 151
- 1. Mineralocorticoids: 151
- 2. Glucocorticoids: 152
- 3. Androgens: 152

8.3 Regulation of Adrenal Cortex Hormone Secretion: 153
- Regulation of Mineralocorticoids: 153
- Regulation of Glucocorticoids: 154
- Regulation of Androgens: 154

8.4 Disorders of the Adrenal Cortex: 155
- Addison's Disease (Primary Adrenal Insufficiency): 155
- Secondary Adrenal Insufficiency: 156
- Cushing's Syndrome: 156
- Hyperaldosteronism: 157

8.5 Conclusion 158

Case Studies 158
- Case Study 1: Addison's Disease 158
- Case Study 2: Cushing's Syndrome 160

Practice Questions for Self-Assessment 161
- Multiple Choice Questions 161
- True or False Questions 163

Answers 163
- Case Study 1 163
- Case Study 2 164
- Multiple Choice Questions 164
- Short Answer Questions 165

True or False Questions 165

Bibliography 166

Chapter Nine 168

9.1 Anatomy and Structure of the Adrenal Medulla 168

Embryological Development and Morphological Features: 168

Microscopic Anatomy: 168

Chromaffin Cells and Innervation: 169

Vasculature and Blood Supply: 169

Extracellular Matrix and Supportive Structures: 169

9.2 Adrenaline and Noradrenaline: Synthesis, Secretion, and Regulation 170

Anatomy and Structure of the Adrenal Medulla: 170

Synthesis Pathway of Adrenaline and Noradrenaline: 170

Secretion Mechanism of Adrenaline and Noradrenaline: 170

Regulation of Synthesis and Secretion: 171

Physiological Effects of Adrenaline and Noradrenaline: 171

9.3 Functions of Adrenal Medulla Hormones: Adrenaline and Noradrenaline 172

Cardiovascular Effects of Adrenal Medulla Hormones: 172

Respiratory Effects of Adrenal Medulla Hormones: 172

Metabolic Effects of Adrenal Medulla Hormones: 173

Effects on Blood Flow Distribution: 173

Pupillary and Central Nervous System Effects: 174

Glycogenolysis and Gluconeogenesis: 174

9.4 Regulation of Adrenal Medulla Hormone Secretion: A Comprehensive Overview 174

Neural Regulation of Adrenal Medulla Hormone Secretion: 175

Neural Inputs Modulating Adrenal Medulla Activity: 175

Hormonal Regulation of Adrenal Medulla Hormone Secretion: 175

Feedback Mechanisms in Adrenal Medulla Regulation: 176

- Circadian Regulation of Adrenal Medulla Activity: 176
- Case Studies 177
  - Case Study 1: Pheochromocytoma and Catecholamine Hypersecretion 177
  - Case Study 2: Chronic Stress and Adrenal Medulla Hyperactivity 178
- Practice Questions for Self-Assessment 180
  - Multiple Choice Questions 180
  - Short Answer Questions 181
  - True or False Questions 181
- Answers 182
  - Case Study 1 182
  - Case Study 2 182
  - Multiple Choice Questions 183
  - Short Answer Questions 183
  - True or False Questions 184
- Bibliography 184
- Chapter 10 187
  - 10.1 Islets of Langerhans: Composition and Functions: 187
    - Composition of Islets of Langerhans 187
    - Functions of Islets of Langerhans 188
    - Clinical Implications and Pathophysiology 189
  - 10.2 Insulin: Synthesis, Secretion, and Actions 190
    - Synthesis of Insulin: 190
    - Secretion of Insulin: 191
    - Actions of Insulin: 191
    - Clinical Relevance: 193
  - 10.3 Glucagon: Synthesis, Secretion, and Actions: 194
    - Synthesis and Secretion: 194

Actions of Glucagon: 194

Regulation of Glucagon Secretion: 195

Clinical Significance: 196

10.4 Regulation of Blood Glucose Levels: A Comprehensive Exploration of Physiological Mechanisms and Clinical Implications: 196

Fed State Regulation: 196

Fasting State Regulation: 197

Counterregulatory Hormones: 198

Neural Regulation: 199

Clinical Implications: 200

10.5 Conclusion: 200

Case Studies 201

Case Study 1: Insulin Deficiency and Diabetes Mellitus 201

Case Study 2: Hypoglycemia in a Type 1 Diabetic Patient 202

Practice Questions for Self-Assessment 204

Multiple Choice Questions 204

Short Answer Questions 205

True or False Questions 205

Answers 205

Case Study 1 205

Case Study 2 206

Multiple Choice Questions 207

Short Answer Questions 207

True or False Questions 208

Bibliography 208

Chapter 11 211

11.1 Anatomy and Histology of Parathyroid Glands: Exploring the Endocrine Regulators of Calcium Homeostasis 211

Anatomy of Parathyroid Glands: 211

Histology of Parathyroid Glands: 211

Functional Significance: 212

11.2 Parathyroid Hormone (PTH): Synthesis, Secretion, and Actions 212

Synthesis and Secretion: 212

Actions of PTH: 213

Regulation of PTH Secretion: 214

Clinical Relevance: 215

11.3 Regulation of Calcium and Phosphate Homeostasis Comprehensive Overview 215

Parathyroid Hormone (PTH): 216

Calcitonin: 216

Vitamin D (Calcitriol): 217

Other Factors: 217

Regulation and Feedback Loops: 218

11.4 Disorders of Parathyroid Glands and Calcium Metabolism 218

Primary Hyperparathyroidism 218

Secondary Hyperparathyroidism 219

Hypoparathyroidism 221

Familial Hypocalciuric Hypercalcemia (FHH) 222

Pseudohypoparathyroidism 222

11.4 Conclusion: 223

Case Studies 224

Case Study 1: Hyperparathyroidism and Hypercalcemia 224

Case Study 2: Hypoparathyroidism and Hypocalcemia 226

Practice Questions for Self-Assessment 227

Multiple Choice Questions 227

Short Answer Questions 229

True or False Questions	229
Answers	230
Case Study 1	230
Case Study 2	230
Multiple Choice Questions	231
Short Answer Questions	231
True or False Questions	232
Bibliography	233
Glossary of Key Terms	234
A	234
B	234
C	234
D	234
E	234
F	235
G	235
H	235
I	235
J	235
K	235
L	235
M	236
N	236
O	236
P	236
R	236
S	236

T	237
U	237
V	237
W	237
X	237
Y	237
Z	237
Books in the same series	238

Dedication

This book is dedicated to all students, researchers, and healthcare professionals who seek to unravel the intricate workings of the endocrine system. May your passion for understanding physiology led to advancements that benefit humankind's health and well-being.

Special gratitude to our families and mentors whose unwavering support and guidance have been instrumental in our journey of learning and discovery.

Preface

Endocrine physiology is a captivating field that lies at the heart of understanding how the body maintains homeostasis and responds to internal and external stimuli. The endocrine system, with its intricate network of glands and hormones, orchestrates a multitude of physiological processes that are essential for growth, metabolism, reproduction, and overall well-being. This book, "Advanced Endocrine Physiology: A Comprehensive Review," is designed to provide a thorough and detailed exploration of this fascinating domain.

The motivation for writing this book stems from a recognition of the critical importance of endocrine physiology in both clinical and research settings. As a human physiologist, I have witnessed firsthand the profound impact that a solid understanding of endocrine mechanisms can have on diagnosing, managing, and treating a wide range of medical conditions. It is my hope that this book will serve as a valuable resource for students, researchers, and healthcare professionals who seek to deepen their knowledge and enhance their practice in this field.

This book is structured to guide readers through the foundational principles of endocrinology, the methods of hormonal assay, and the detailed physiology of key endocrine organs and systems. Each chapter is meticulously crafted to provide clear explanations, supported by diagrams, clinical correlations, and the latest research findings. The aim is to make complex concepts accessible and to encourage the application of this knowledge in various contexts.

In the pages that follow, you will find a comprehensive review of topics ranging from the physiology of the hypothalamus and pituitary gland to the regulation of growth, thyroid function, adrenal physiology, glucose metabolism, and calcium homeostasis. Special attention is given to the mechanisms of hormonal action and the feedback loops that maintain endocrine balance. Additionally, the appendices offer practical resources such as a glossary of key terms, diagrams of hormonal pathways, and self-assessment questions to reinforce learning.

The field of endocrinology is dynamic, with continuous advancements and discoveries. Therefore, this book also looks toward the future, highlighting emerging trends and potential directions for research. My goal is to equip readers with a solid foundation in endocrine physiology while inspiring curiosity and a lifelong pursuit of knowledge in this ever-evolving discipline.

I extend my gratitude to colleagues, mentors, and students who have contributed their insights and feedback during the development of this book. Their contributions have been invaluable in shaping its content and ensuring its relevance and accuracy.

It is with great enthusiasm that I present "Advanced Endocrine Physiology: A Comprehensive Review." May it serve as a comprehensive guide and an enduring reference for all who seek to understand and advance the science of endocrine physiology.

Professor Gideon A.G (PhD)

Chapter 1

Principles of Endocrinology

1.1 Introduction to Endocrinology

Endocrinology is a branch of biology and medicine that deals with the study of hormones, their synthesis, secretion, mechanisms of action, and physiological effects on target tissues. Hormones are signaling molecules produced by specialized cells or glands in the body, known as endocrine glands, and they play pivotal roles in regulating numerous physiological processes, including metabolism, growth and development, reproduction, immune function, and response to stress. The history of endocrinology dates back to the 19th century when scientists began to recognize the importance of glands in secreting substances that regulate bodily functions. One of the landmark discoveries in endocrinology was made by Thomas Addison in 1855 when he described the clinical manifestations of adrenal insufficiency, now known as Addison's disease, highlighting the critical role of the adrenal glands in maintaining health.

The term "endocrinology" was coined by Ernest Starling in 1905, derived from the Greek words "Endon," meaning within, and "kinesin," meaning to secrete. This reflects the focus of endocrinology on the study of internal secretions, or hormones, which are released directly into the bloodstream to exert their effects on distant target cells or tissues.

Endocrinology encompasses a wide range of hormones, including peptides, steroids, amines, and fatty acid derivatives, each with unique chemical structures and mechanisms of action. Peptide hormones, such as insulin and growth hormone, are synthesized as prohormones and processed into active forms before being secreted into the bloodstream. Steroid hormones, such as cortisol and estrogen, are derived from cholesterol and are synthesized and released by endocrine glands such as the adrenal cortex and gonads.

The endocrine system is composed of various glands distributed throughout the body, including the pituitary gland, thyroid gland, adrenal glands, pancreas, and gonads, as well as numerous other tissues and organs that produce hormones locally. These glands work in concert to maintain homeostasis by coordinating physiological responses to internal and external stimuli.

Advances in molecular biology, genetics, and biochemistry have revolutionized our understanding of endocrine physiology and the pathophysiology of endocrine disorders. Techniques such as gene cloning, recombinant DNA technology, and molecular imaging have provided insights into the molecular mechanisms underlying hormone synthesis, secretion, and action, as well as the development of targeted therapies for endocrine disorders.

1.2 Hormones: Definition, Classification, and Functions

Hormones are signaling molecules produced by specialized cells or glands in the body, collectively known as endocrine glands. These molecules are released into the bloodstream and carried to target tissues or organs, where they exert their physiological effects by binding to specific receptors.

Classification of Hormones:

Hormones can be classified into several categories based on their chemical structure, mode of action, and site of synthesis.

1. Peptide Hormones:

- Definition: Peptide hormones are composed of short chains of amino acids.

- Examples: Insulin, glucagon, growth hormone (GH), prolactin, parathyroid hormone (PTH), adrenocorticotropic hormone (ACTH).

- Characteristics: Peptide hormones are water-soluble and typically act on cell surface receptors. They exert their effects by initiating intracellular signaling cascades through second messenger systems such as cyclic adenosine monophosphate (cAMP) or calcium ions.

2. Steroid Hormones:

- Definition: Steroid hormones are derived from cholesterol.

- Examples: Cortisol, aldosterone, estrogen, progesterone, testosterone.

- Characteristics: Steroid hormones are lipid-soluble and can diffuse across cell membranes. They bind to intracellular receptors, modulating gene expression and protein synthesis.

3. Amino Acid-Derived Hormones:

- Definition: Amino acid-derived hormones are synthesized from amino acids.

- Examples: Thyroid hormones (T3 and T4), catecholamines (epinephrine, norepinephrine).

- Characteristics: Thyroid hormones act intracellularly like steroids, while catecholamines primarily act through cell surface receptors.

4. Fatty Acid-Derived Hormones:

- Definition: Fatty acid-derived hormones are derived from fatty acids.

- Examples: Eicosanoids (prostaglandins, leukotrienes).

- Characteristics: Eicosanoids exert localized effects as autocrine or paracrine signaling molecules, influencing inflammation, blood clotting, and smooth muscle contraction.

5. Gaseous Hormones:

- Definition: Gaseous hormones are small, volatile molecules that act as signaling molecules.

- Examples: Nitric oxide (NO), carbon monoxide (CO).

- Characteristics: Gaseous hormones exert their effects by diffusing through cell membranes and modulating intracellular signaling pathways.

6. Peptide Hormones with Cyclic Structure:

  - Definition: Peptide hormones with cyclic structure contain additional bonds between amino acids, forming cyclic peptides.

  - Examples: Oxytocin, vasopressin (antidiuretic hormone, ADH).

  - Characteristics: These hormones often have specific roles in regulating reproductive functions, water balance, and blood pressure.

7. Neurohormones:

  - Definition: Neurohormones are hormones produced by neurons and released into the bloodstream.

  - Examples: Hypothalamic hormones (e.g., gonadotropin-releasing hormone, GnRH), catecholamines (epinephrine, norepinephrine) released from the adrenal medulla.

  - Characteristics: Neurohormones play crucial roles in regulating physiological processes, including stress response, reproduction, and metabolism.

Functions of Hormones:

Hormones play diverse and essential roles in regulating numerous physiological processes throughout the body. Some of the key functions of hormones include:

1. Metabolism Regulation: Hormones such as insulin, glucagon, thyroid hormones (T3 and T4), and cortisol play pivotal roles in regulating metabolism. They control the breakdown, utilization, and storage of carbohydrates, fats, and proteins, influencing energy production and nutrient utilization.

2. Growth and Development: Growth hormone (GH), insulin-like growth factors (IGFs), and thyroid hormones are crucial for normal growth and development, particularly during childhood and adolescence. They stimulate cell proliferation, differentiation, and growth of tissues, bones, and organs.

3. Reproductive Function: Sex hormones, including estrogen, progesterone, and testosterone, regulate reproductive processes such as gametogenesis (sperm and egg production), sexual differentiation, and the menstrual cycle. They also influence secondary sexual characteristics and fertility.

4. Stress Response: Hormones such as cortisol (produced by the adrenal cortex) and epinephrine (adrenaline, produced by the adrenal medulla) mediate the body's response to stress. They mobilize energy reserves, increase heart rate and blood pressure, and redirect blood flow to vital organs during fight-or-flight responses.

5. Fluid and Electrolyte Balance: Hormones like aldosterone (produced by the adrenal cortex) and antidiuretic hormone (ADH, produced by the hypothalamus and released by the posterior pituitary gland) regulate water and electrolyte balance by influencing renal reabsorption and excretion.

6. Blood Pressure Regulation: Hormones such as renin, aldosterone, and natriuretic peptides regulate blood pressure by modulating blood volume, vascular tone, and renal function. They help maintain systemic blood pressure within a narrow range to ensure adequate perfusion of tissues and organs.

7. Bone Metabolism: Hormones like parathyroid hormone (PTH) and calcitonin regulate calcium and phosphate homeostasis, influencing bone formation, resorption, and mineralization. They help maintain skeletal integrity and electrolyte balance.

8. Immune Function: Some hormones, including cytokines (such as interleukins and interferons) and thymosin (produced by the thymus gland), modulate immune cell function and inflammation. They regulate the immune response to pathogens, allergens, and foreign antigens, contributing to the body's defense mechanisms.

9. Circadian Rhythms: Hormones such as melatonin (produced by the pineal gland) and cortisol (regulated by the hypothalamus-pituitary-adrenal axis) help regulate circadian rhythms, including sleep-wake cycles, body temperature, and hormonal secretion patterns.

10. Mood and Behavior: Neurotransmitter-like hormones, such as serotonin and dopamine, influence mood, cognition, and behavior. They play roles in regulating emotions, motivation, reward pathways, and stress resilience.

1.3 Mechanisms of Hormone Action

Hormones exert their effects on target cells through various mechanisms, depending on their chemical nature and the location of their receptors. The two primary mechanisms of hormone action are via cell surface receptors (for water-soluble hormones) and intracellular receptors (for lipid-soluble hormones).

Cell Surface Receptors:

Cell surface receptors, also known as membrane receptors, are integral membrane proteins located on the plasma membrane of target cells. They play a crucial role in mediating the effects of water-soluble hormones, such as peptide hormones and catecholamines. The interaction between these hormones and their respective receptors initiates intracellular signaling cascades, leading to various cellular responses. Several types of cell surface receptors are involved in hormone action, including G protein-coupled receptors (GPCRs) and receptor tyrosine kinases (RTKs).

G Protein-Coupled Receptors (GPCRs):

G protein-coupled receptors (GPCRs) represent the largest family of cell surface receptors involved in signal transduction. They play a pivotal role in mediating the effects of numerous hormones, neurotransmitters, and sensory stimuli on cellular function. The structure, signaling pathways, and physiological roles of GPCRs are diverse and intricate.

Structure of GPCRs:

- GPCRs are integral membrane proteins composed of seven transmembrane helices connected by intra- and extracellular loops.

- The N-terminus of the receptor is located extracellularly, while the C-terminus is intracellular.

- Ligand binding occurs at the extracellular domain, leading to conformational changes that activate the receptor.

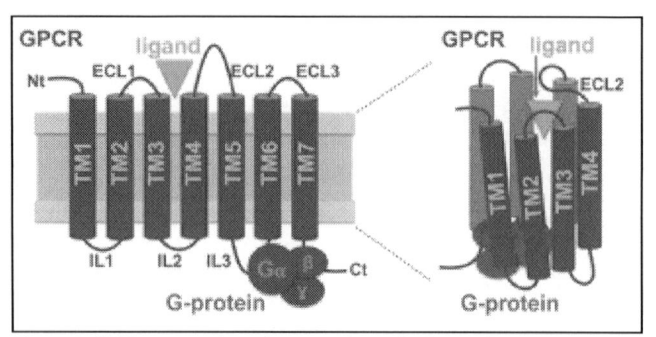

Figure 1: GPCRs, a type of membrane protein, are fundamentally structured with seven helices that span across the membrane. These helices are linked together by loops, some of which are situated inside the cell (intracellular loops), and others that are located outside the cell (extracellular loops).

Signaling Pathways:

- Activation of GPCRs triggers a cascade of intracellular signaling events mediated by heterotrimeric G proteins.

- G proteins consist of α, β, and γ subunits, with the α subunit being the primary effector of signaling.

- Ligand binding induces a conformational change in the receptor, promoting the exchange of GDP for GTP on the α subunit, leading to its dissociation from the βγ subunits.

- Both the α-GTP and βγ subunits can modulate the activity of downstream effector molecules, such as adenylyl cyclase, phospholipase C (PLC), and ion channels.

- Adenylyl cyclase activation leads to the production of cyclic adenosine monophosphate (cAMP), which serves as a second messenger in various cellular processes.

- PLC activation results in the hydrolysis of phosphatidylinositol 4,5-bisphosphate (PIP2) into inositol trisphosphate (IP3) and diacylglycerol (DAG), leading to calcium release from intracellular stores and activation of protein kinase C (PKC).

- GPCR-mediated signaling pathways modulate cellular responses such as gene transcription, neurotransmitter release, ion channel activity, and cytoskeletal rearrangements.

Physiological Roles:

- GPCRs regulate a wide range of physiological processes, including neurotransmission, hormone secretion, sensory perception, and immune response.

- Examples of GPCR-mediated signaling pathways include the β-adrenergic receptor pathway, involved in the regulation of heart rate and contractility, and the muscarinic acetylcholine receptor pathway, mediating parasympathetic neurotransmission.

- Dysregulation of GPCR signaling has been implicated in various diseases, including cardiovascular disorders, neurodegenerative diseases, and cancer, making GPCRs attractive targets for drug development.

Receptor Tyrosine Kinases (RTKs):

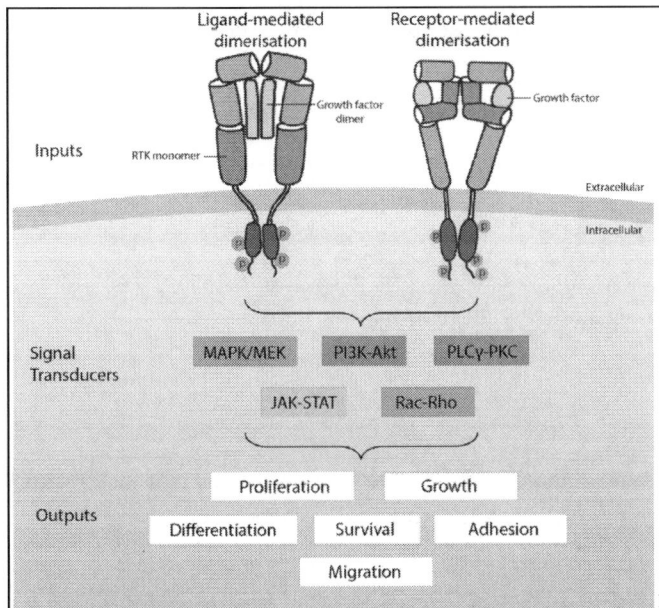

Figure 2: provides a broad summary of the activation, signaling, and subsequent cellular decisions influenced by receptor tyrosine kinases. The process begins when growth factors (inputs) in the extracellular environment bind to the receptor, causing a change in its structure that allows dimerization. This leads to autophosphorylation (indicated by circled p) by the intracellular tyrosine kinase domains, resulting in the recruitment of one or more signal transduction pathways. These pathways then transmit the signal to effectors that ultimately determine cell fates (outputs). The pathways involved include mitogen-activated protein kinase (MAPK), phosphatidylinositol 3-kinase–protein kinase B (PI3K–Akt), phospholipase C gamma–protein kinase C (PLCgamma–PKC), and Janus kinase and signal transducer and activator of transcription (JAK–STAT).

- RTKs are a family of cell surface receptors characterized by an intracellular tyrosine kinase domain that phosphorylates tyrosine residues on target proteins.

- Structure: RTKs typically consist of an extracellular ligand-binding domain, a single transmembrane domain, and an intracellular tyrosine kinase domain.

- Activation: Binding of the hormone to the extracellular domain of the RTK induces receptor dimerization or oligomerization, leading to autophosphorylation of tyrosine residues in the intracellular domain.

- Signal Transduction: Phosphorylated tyrosine residues on the RTK serve as docking sites for intracellular signaling proteins, such as adaptor proteins and enzymes, which propagate the hormonal signal. Activation of RTKs can lead to the activation of various downstream pathways, including the Ras/mitogen-activated protein kinase (MAPK) pathway, the phosphoinositide 3-kinase (PI3K)/Akt pathway, and the Janus kinase/signal transducer and activator of transcription (JAK/STAT) pathway.

- Examples: The insulin receptor, a prototypical RTK, binds insulin and activates downstream signaling pathways involved in glucose uptake, glycogen synthesis, and gene expression. The epidermal growth factor receptor (EGFR), another RTK, mediates cellular responses to growth factors and regulates cell proliferation, differentiation, and survival.

Intracellular Receptors:

Intracellular receptors play a vital role in mediating the actions of lipid-soluble hormones, such as steroid hormones and thyroid hormones. These receptors are located inside the cell, either in the cytoplasm or nucleus, and upon hormone binding, they initiate a cascade of events that regulate gene expression and protein synthesis.

1. Ligand Binding and Receptor Activation:

- Lipid-soluble hormones, including steroid hormones (e.g., cortisol, estrogen, testosterone) and thyroid hormones (T3 and T4), can diffuse across cell membranes due to their hydrophobic nature.

- Once inside the cell, these hormones bind to specific intracellular receptors, forming hormone-receptor complexes.

- The binding of the hormone induces a conformational change in the receptor, exposing nuclear localization signals and/or DNA-binding domains, which are essential for their transcriptional regulatory functions.

2. Translocation to the Nucleus:

- The hormone-receptor complex translocates to the nucleus, facilitated by nuclear localization signals present on the receptor or associated chaperone proteins.

- In the case of steroid hormones, the receptor is often bound to heat shock proteins (HSPs) in the cytoplasm, which dissociate upon hormone binding, allowing the receptor to translocate to the nucleus.

3. DNA Binding and Gene Regulation:

- Once inside the nucleus, the hormone-receptor complex binds to specific DNA sequences called hormone response elements (HREs) located in the promoter regions of target genes.

- The binding of the hormone-receptor complex to HREs modulates the transcription of target genes, either by promoting gene expression (transactivation) or repressing gene transcription (transrepression).

- This transcriptional regulation leads to the synthesis of new mRNA transcripts, which are subsequently translated into proteins that mediate the biological effects of the hormone.

4. Coactivators and Corepressors:

- Intracellular receptors often interact with coactivator or corepressor proteins, which influence their transcriptional activity.

- Coactivators enhance the transcriptional activity of the hormone-receptor complex by facilitating chromatin remodeling, recruitment of RNA polymerase, and assembly of transcriptional machinery.

- Corepressors, on the other hand, suppress gene transcription by promoting chromatin condensation or inhibiting the recruitment of transcriptional activators.

5. Gene Expression and Protein Synthesis:

- The transcriptional regulation mediated by intracellular receptors leads to changes in gene expression, resulting in the synthesis of specific proteins within the target cell.

- These proteins may include enzymes, structural proteins, or regulatory factors that mediate the physiological effects of the hormone, such as metabolic enzymes, cell signaling molecules, or transcription factors.

6. Physiological Effects:

- The ultimate physiological effects of intracellular receptor-mediated hormone action are diverse and depend on the target tissue, the specific genes regulated by the hormone, and the cellular context.

- For example, steroid hormones regulate various physiological processes, including metabolism, immune function, reproductive function, and stress response, by modulating gene expression in target cells.

Nuclear Receptors:

Nuclear receptors are a class of intracellular receptors that play a crucial role in mediating the effects of lipid-soluble hormones, including steroid hormones and thyroid hormones. These receptors function as ligand-activated transcription factors, modulating gene expression in response to hormone binding. The following elucidates the key aspects of nuclear receptors:

Structure of Nuclear Receptors:

- Nuclear receptors typically consist of several functional domains, including a ligand-binding domain (LBD), a DNA-binding domain (DBD), and transcriptional activation domains (AF-1 and AF-2).

- The ligand-binding domain is responsible for hormone binding and undergoes conformational changes upon ligand binding, facilitating receptor activation.

- The DNA-binding domain recognizes specific DNA sequences known as hormone response elements (HREs) located in the promoter regions of target genes.

Mechanism of Action:

- In the absence of hormone binding, nuclear receptors are often associated with co-repressor proteins, maintaining the receptor in an inactive state.

- Upon hormone binding, nuclear receptors undergo a conformational change that promotes dissociation of co-repressor proteins and recruitment of co-activator proteins.

- The hormone-receptor-co-activator complex then binds to HREs in the promoter regions of target genes, leading to transcriptional activation or repression.

- This process results in the modulation of gene expression, ultimately influencing cellular functions and physiological responses.

Examples of Nuclear Receptors:

1. Glucocorticoid Receptor (GR): Activated by glucocorticoid hormones such as cortisol, the glucocorticoid receptor regulates gene expression involved in metabolism, inflammation, and stress response.

2. Estrogen Receptor (ER): Estrogen receptors are activated by estrogen hormones and play essential roles in reproductive physiology, bone metabolism, and cardiovascular health.

3. Androgen Receptor (AR): The androgen receptor mediates the effects of androgen hormones such as testosterone, regulating gene expression related to sexual development, muscle growth, and bone density.

4. Thyroid Hormone Receptor (TR): Thyroid hormone receptors respond to thyroid hormones (T3 and T4) and modulate gene expression involved in metabolism, growth, and development.

Physiological Significance:

- Nuclear receptors play critical roles in various physiological processes, including metabolism, growth, development, reproduction, and immune function.

- Dysregulation of nuclear receptor signaling pathways can lead to a wide range of disorders, including metabolic syndrome, cancer, and autoimmune diseases.

- Pharmacological modulation of nuclear receptor activity is a common therapeutic strategy for managing hormone-related conditions, such as hormone replacement therapy and treatment of endocrine disorders.

1.4 Regulation of Hormone Secretion

Hormone secretion is intricately regulated by a complex interplay of neural, hormonal, and environmental factors to maintain physiological homeostasis. The hypothalamus-pituitary axis serves as the central regulator of hormone secretion, orchestrating the release of hormones from various endocrine glands throughout the body.

Hypothalamus-Pituitary Axis

The hypothalamus-pituitary axis (HPA) is a vital neuroendocrine system that regulates the secretion of hormones from the pituitary gland, thereby controlling numerous physiological processes throughout the body. This axis represents a critical link between the nervous and endocrine systems, allowing the brain to communicate with peripheral glands and organs via hormonal signaling.

Anatomy and Functional Anatomy:

The HPA axis comprises the hypothalamus, the pituitary gland, and their intricate connections. The hypothalamus, a small region located at the base of the brain, serves as the primary control center for the endocrine system. It integrates signals from various regions of the brain and responds to internal and external stimuli to regulate hormone secretion.

The hypothalamus communicates with the pituitary gland via the pituitary stalk (also known as the infundibulum) and the hypophyseal portal system, a network of blood vessels that carries hypothalamic hormones to the anterior pituitary. The posterior pituitary, on the other hand, is a direct extension of the hypothalamus, with neurons projecting from the hypothalamus to release neurohormones into the bloodstream.

Regulation of Hormone Secretion:

The hypothalamus produces a variety of releasing and inhibiting hormones that control the secretion of pituitary hormones. These hypothalamic hormones are secreted into the hypophyseal portal system and reach the anterior pituitary, where they exert their effects on specific cell types.

For example, thyrotropin-releasing hormone (TRH) stimulates the release of thyroid-stimulating hormone (TSH) from thyrotroph cells in the anterior pituitary. Similarly, corticotropin-releasing hormone (CRH) stimulates the secretion of adrenocorticotropic hormone (ACTH) from corticotroph cells, while gonadotropin-releasing hormone (GnRH) regulates the release of luteinizing hormone (LH) and follicle-stimulating hormone (FSH) from gonadotroph cells.

Feedback Regulation:

The secretion of hypothalamic releasing and inhibiting hormones is tightly regulated by feedback mechanisms to maintain hormonal balance. Negative feedback loops play a crucial role in this regulation, where elevated levels of peripheral hormones inhibit the secretion of hypothalamic releasing hormones, thereby reducing pituitary hormone release.

For example, elevated levels of cortisol inhibit the secretion of CRH and ACTH via negative feedback, thereby modulating the stress response. Similarly, high levels of thyroid hormones inhibit the secretion of TRH and TSH, regulating thyroid function.

Integration with Physiological Processes:

The HPA axis is intricately involved in regulating numerous physiological processes, including stress response, growth and development, metabolism, reproduction, and immune function. Dysregulation of the HPA axis can lead to various endocrine disorders, such as Cushing's syndrome, Addison's disease, and hypopituitarism.

Releasing and Inhibiting Factors

The regulation of hormone secretion within the endocrine system involves a sophisticated interplay of releasing and inhibiting factors, which are produced by the hypothalamus and act on the anterior pituitary gland to modulate the release of specific tropic hormones. These tropic hormones, in turn, stimulate or inhibit the activity of target endocrine glands, resulting in the secretion of their respective hormones.

Releasing Factors:

Releasing factors are hormones produced by the hypothalamus that stimulate the secretion of tropic hormones from the anterior pituitary gland. These factors travel through the hypophyseal portal system, a specialized network of blood vessels that connects the hypothalamus to the anterior pituitary, allowing for direct communication between these two structures. Upon reaching the anterior pituitary, releasing factors bind to specific receptors on pituitary cells, triggering intracellular signaling cascades that culminate in the synthesis and release of tropic hormones into the bloodstream.

Examples of releasing factors include:

- Thyrotropin-releasing hormone (TRH): Stimulates the secretion of thyroid-stimulating hormone (TSH) from the anterior pituitary, which, in turn, stimulates the thyroid gland to produce thyroid hormones (T3 and T4).

- Gonadotropin-releasing hormone (GnRH): Stimulates the secretion of luteinizing hormone (LH) and follicle-stimulating hormone (FSH) from the anterior pituitary, which regulate the function of the gonads (testes and ovaries) and the production of sex hormones (testosterone and estrogen).

- Growth hormone-releasing hormone (GHRH): Stimulates the secretion of growth hormone (GH) from the anterior pituitary, which promotes growth and metabolism.

Inhibiting Factors:

Inhibiting factors, also known as inhibitory hormones or factors, are hormones produced by the hypothalamus that suppress the secretion of tropic hormones from the anterior pituitary gland. Similar to releasing factors, inhibiting factors are transported to the anterior pituitary via the hypophyseal portal system, where they exert their inhibitory effects on pituitary cells.

Examples of inhibiting factors include:

- Somatostatin (also known as growth hormone-inhibiting hormone, GHIH): Inhibits the secretion of growth hormone (GH) from the anterior pituitary, counteracting the effects of growth hormone-releasing hormone (GHRH).

- Dopamine (also known as prolactin-inhibiting hormone, PIH): Inhibits the secretion of prolactin (PRL) from the anterior pituitary, regulating lactation and reproductive function.

- Corticotropin-inhibiting hormone (CIH): Inhibits the secretion of adrenocorticotropic hormone (ACTH) from the anterior pituitary, modulating the body's response to stress and inflammation.

The balance between releasing and inhibiting factors is crucial for maintaining hormonal homeostasis and ensuring proper physiological function. Dysregulation of these factors can lead to the development of endocrine disorders, such as hypothyroidism, hyperthyroidism, or hypogonadism. Further research into the mechanisms underlying the action of releasing and inhibiting factors is essential for advancing our understanding of endocrine physiology and developing targeted therapies for endocrine-related diseases.

Negative Feedback

Negative feedback is a fundamental regulatory mechanism in the endocrine system that helps maintain hormone levels within a narrow physiological range. It operates through a self-regulating loop wherein the output of a system acts to inhibit or reduce the activity of the system itself. In the context of hormone secretion, negative feedback mechanisms ensure that hormone levels remain balanced and prevent excessive stimulation or inhibition of endocrine glands.

Key Components of Negative Feedback Loop:

1. Sensor: The sensor detects changes in hormone levels and sends signals to the control center.

2. Control Center: In the endocrine system, the control center typically refers to the hypothalamus or pituitary gland, which receives input from the sensor and regulates hormone secretion accordingly.

3. Effector: The effector is the endocrine gland that produces and releases the hormone in response to signals from the control center.

4. Feedback Signal: The feedback signal is the hormone itself or another molecule that inhibits hormone secretion when levels exceed a certain threshold.

Mechanism of Negative Feedback Loop:

1. Stimulus: The negative feedback loop begins with a stimulus that disrupts homeostasis, such as a decrease or increase in hormone levels.

2. Detection: Sensors in the body detect the change in hormone levels and transmit this information to the control center.

3. Control Center Response: The control center, typically the hypothalamus or pituitary gland, responds to the detected change by releasing signaling molecules (e.g., releasing hormones or inhibiting hormones) to regulate hormone secretion from the effector gland.

4. Effector Response: The effector gland, in response to the signals from the control center, adjusts its hormone secretion accordingly. If hormone levels are too high, secretion may be inhibited, whereas if levels are too low, secretion may be stimulated.

5. Feedback Inhibition: Once hormone levels return to within the normal range, the feedback signal acts to inhibit further secretion from the effector gland, closing the loop and restoring homeostasis.

Examples of Negative Feedback in Endocrine System:

- Thyroid Hormone Regulation: High levels of thyroid hormones inhibit the release of thyroid-stimulating hormone (TSH) from the anterior pituitary gland. Conversely, low levels of thyroid hormones stimulate TSH secretion, leading to increased thyroid hormone production.

- Cortisol Regulation: Cortisol, a stress hormone produced by the adrenal glands, inhibits the release of adrenocorticotropic hormone (ACTH) from the pituitary gland when levels are elevated. This negative feedback loop helps regulate cortisol secretion in response to stress.

Negative feedback mechanisms are crucial for maintaining hormonal balance and preventing overactivity or underactivity of endocrine glands. Dysregulation of these feedback loops can lead to hormonal imbalances and contribute to the development of endocrine disorders such as hyperthyroidism, hypothyroidism, and Cushing's syndrome.

Circadian Rhythms and Environmental Cues

The endocrine system exhibits rhythmic variations in hormone secretion, known as circadian rhythms, which are synchronized with the light-dark cycle of the environment. These rhythms are regulated by internal biological clocks located in the suprachiasmatic nucleus (SCN) of the hypothalamus and are influenced by external environmental cues, such as light exposure, temperature, and feeding-fasting cycles.

Suprachiasmatic Nucleus (SCN):

The SCN serves as the master circadian pacemaker, coordinating the body's internal rhythms with external environmental cues. Neurons within the SCN contain intrinsic molecular clocks that generate self-sustained oscillations with a period of approximately 24 hours. These clocks are synchronized, or entrained, to the external light-dark cycle through input from the retinohypothalamic tract, which relays information about light exposure directly from the retina to the SCN.

Light-Dark Cycle:

Light is the most potent environmental cue for entraining circadian rhythms. Exposure to light during the day suppresses the production of melatonin, a hormone synthesized and released by the pineal gland that regulates sleep-wake cycles. As night falls and light levels decrease, melatonin secretion increases, promoting sleep and synchronizing circadian rhythms with the dark phase of the day-night cycle.

Temperature and Feeding-Fasting Cycles:

In addition to light, other environmental cues, such as temperature and feeding-fasting cycles, also influence circadian rhythms. Body temperature exhibits a circadian rhythm, with a nadir during the early morning hours and a peak in the late afternoon or early evening. Feeding and fasting cycles, regulated by hormones such as insulin and ghrelin, can also affect circadian rhythms, particularly in peripheral tissues involved in metabolism.

Endocrine Regulation of Circadian Rhythms:

The circadian timing system exerts profound effects on the endocrine system, regulating the timing and amplitude of hormone secretion. Many hormones, including cortisol, growth hormone, and thyroid-stimulating hormone, exhibit circadian variation in secretion, with peaks and troughs occurring at specific times of day. These rhythmic fluctuations optimize physiological processes to align with the body's changing metabolic and behavioral demands throughout the day.

Clinical Implications:

Disruptions to circadian rhythms, such as shift work, jet lag, or chronic sleep disturbances, can have detrimental effects on health and well-being. Circadian misalignment has been linked to an increased risk of metabolic disorders, cardiovascular disease, mood disorders, and impaired immune function.

Stress Response

The stress response is a fundamental adaptive mechanism that enables organisms to cope with challenging or threatening situations. The endocrine system plays a pivotal role in orchestrating the body's response to stress, primarily through the activation of the hypothalamic-pituitary-adrenal (HPA) axis.

Activation of the HPA Axis

When the body perceives a stressor, whether physical, psychological, or environmental, the hypothalamus responds by releasing corticotropin-releasing hormone (CRH) into the hypophyseal portal system. CRH then stimulates the anterior pituitary gland to secrete adrenocorticotropic hormone (ACTH) into the bloodstream.

Release of Cortisol

ACTH, in turn, stimulates the adrenal cortex to produce and release cortisol, a glucocorticoid hormone. Cortisol exerts a multitude of effects throughout the body to prepare it to cope with the stressor. These effects include:

- Metabolic Response: Cortisol increases blood glucose levels by promoting gluconeogenesis (the synthesis of glucose from non-carbohydrate sources) and glycogenolysis (the breakdown of glycogen into glucose). Elevated blood glucose provides additional energy to fuel the body's response to stress.

- Immunosuppressive Effects: Cortisol suppresses the immune system's inflammatory response by inhibiting the production of pro-inflammatory cytokines and reducing the activity of immune cells such as lymphocytes and macrophages. This anti-inflammatory effect helps prevent excessive tissue damage during the stress response.

- Cardiovascular Effects: Cortisol enhances cardiovascular function by increasing heart rate, cardiac output, and vascular tone. These changes facilitate the delivery of oxygen and nutrients to vital organs and tissues, preparing the body for increased physical activity.

- Behavioral and Cognitive Effects: Cortisol influences mood, cognition, and behavior, promoting alertness, arousal, and vigilance during stressful situations. However, chronic elevation of cortisol levels can lead to cognitive impairment, mood disturbances, and anxiety disorders.

Negative Feedback Regulation

Once the stressor has been resolved, cortisol levels return to baseline through negative feedback regulation. Elevated cortisol levels inhibit further release of CRH and ACTH from the hypothalamus and pituitary gland, respectively, shutting down the HPA axis. This feedback loop helps restore homeostasis and prevent prolonged activation of the stress response, which could be detrimental to health if sustained over time.

Dysregulation of the Stress Response

Chronic or excessive activation of the stress response can have detrimental effects on health. Prolonged elevation of cortisol levels, as seen in chronic stress or stress-related disorders, is associated with a range of adverse effects, including metabolic disturbances, immune dysfunction, cardiovascular disease, mood disorders, and cognitive impairment. Understanding the mechanisms underlying the stress response and its regulation is essential for developing interventions to mitigate the negative health consequences of chronic stress.

In summary, the stress response is a complex physiological process involving the activation of the HPA axis and the release of cortisol to mobilize resources and adapt to challenging situations. While acute stress is a normal and adaptive response, chronic or excessive stress can have profound implications for health and well-being. Further research into the mechanisms underlying stress regulation is needed to develop effective strategies for managing stress-related disorders and promoting resilience in the face of adversity.

1.5 Feedback Mechanisms in the Endocrine System

Feedback mechanisms are essential regulatory processes that ensure the maintenance of homeostasis within the endocrine system. These mechanisms involve the detection of changes in hormone levels by various sensors or receptors, which subsequently trigger responses to either amplify or dampen hormone secretion. Two primary types of feedback loops, negative and positive feedback, play crucial roles in modulating hormone secretion and maintaining physiological balance.

Negative Feedback Mechanism:

Negative feedback mechanisms are fundamental regulatory processes within the endocrine system that help maintain homeostasis by counteracting changes in hormone levels. In negative feedback loops, the response to a stimulus opposes the initial change, thereby stabilizing hormone levels within a narrow physiological range. This regulatory mechanism ensures that hormone secretion is neither excessive nor deficient, optimizing physiological function.

Key components of negative feedback mechanisms in the endocrine system include:

1. Stimulus: Negative feedback loops begin with a stimulus that triggers hormone secretion. This stimulus can be internal (e.g., fluctuation in blood glucose levels) or external (e.g., stress).

2. Sensor: Specialized cells or receptors within the body detect changes in hormone levels or other physiological parameters. These sensors provide feedback to the endocrine glands, initiating the regulatory response.

3. Effector: Endocrine glands, such as the hypothalamus, pituitary gland, thyroid gland, adrenal glands, pancreas, and others, act as effectors that produce and secrete hormones in response to the stimulus.

4. Hormone Secretion: In response to the stimulus, the effector gland secretes hormones into the bloodstream. These hormones travel to target tissues or organs, where they exert their physiological effects.

5. Inhibition: As hormone levels rise in the bloodstream, they exert negative feedback effects on the hypothalamus and/or pituitary gland, inhibiting further hormone secretion. This inhibition helps prevent excessive hormone production and maintains hormonal balance.

6. Restoration of Homeostasis: The inhibition of hormone secretion restores homeostasis by reducing the stimulus that initially triggered hormone release. This negative feedback loop helps stabilize hormone levels within the optimal range for physiological function.

Examples of negative feedback mechanisms in the endocrine system include:

- Regulation of thyroid hormone (TH) secretion by the hypothalamic-pituitary-thyroid axis.

- Control of blood glucose levels through insulin and glucagon secretion by the pancreas.

- Regulation of adrenal hormone secretion (e.g., cortisol) in response to stress via the hypothalamic-pituitary-adrenal (HPA) axis.

- Maintenance of calcium homeostasis through parathyroid hormone (PTH) secretion in response to changes in blood calcium levels.

Overall, negative feedback mechanisms play a crucial role in maintaining hormonal balance and ensuring the proper functioning of physiological processes. By modulating hormone secretion in response to changing internal and external conditions, negative feedback loops help preserve homeostasis and support overall health and well-being.

Positive Feedback Mechanism:

Positive feedback mechanisms are regulatory processes within the endocrine system that amplify and reinforce physiological responses to certain stimuli, leading to a cascade of events that ultimately culminate in a specific endpoint. Unlike negative feedback mechanisms, which work to maintain homeostasis by counteracting changes, positive feedback loops intensify the initial stimulus, promoting a rapid and often exponential increase in hormone secretion or physiological activity. While less common than negative feedback, positive feedback plays critical roles in processes such as childbirth, lactation, and certain aspects of hormone regulation.

Key components of positive feedback mechanisms in the endocrine system include:

Stimulus: Positive feedback loops begin with a stimulus that triggers a physiological response. This stimulus initiates a cascade of events that further enhances the original stimulus, leading to an amplification of the response.

Effector: Endocrine glands or other physiological effectors respond to the initial stimulus by secreting hormones or activating other signaling pathways.

Amplification: The effector's response amplifies the initial stimulus, leading to increased hormone secretion or physiological activity.

Continuation: The amplified response further stimulates the effector, creating a self-reinforcing cycle that continues until an external factor intervenes to halt the positive feedback loop.

Endpoint: The positive feedback loop culminates in a specific endpoint or physiological event, at which point the stimulus is removed, and the feedback loop is terminated.

Examples of positive feedback mechanisms in the endocrine system include:

- Childbirth: During labor, uterine contractions stimulate the release of oxytocin from the posterior pituitary gland. Oxytocin, in turn, enhances uterine contractions, leading to further oxytocin release. This positive feedback loop continues until the baby is delivered, at which point the stimulus (pressure on the cervix) is removed, and oxytocin secretion ceases.

- Lactation: After childbirth, suckling by the infant stimulates nerve endings in the nipple, triggering the release of oxytocin from the posterior pituitary gland. Oxytocin causes contraction of the myoepithelial cells surrounding the mammary alveoli, leading to the ejection of milk. The continued suckling and milk removal further stimulate oxytocin release, creating a positive feedback loop that promotes milk production and breastfeeding.

- Gonadotropin Release during Menstrual Cycle: In females, rising levels of estrogen during the menstrual cycle stimulate the release of luteinizing hormone (LH) from the anterior pituitary gland. LH, in turn, triggers ovulation, leading to the release of an egg from the ovary. This positive feedback loop promotes the continuation of the menstrual cycle until ovulation occurs.

1.6 Conclusion

In this chapter, we established the foundational concepts of endocrinology, defining its scope and highlighting the role of hormones in regulating numerous physiological processes. We examined the classification of hormones and the mechanisms of their action, emphasizing the importance of receptor interactions and intracellular signaling pathways.

We also explored the regulatory mechanisms that maintain hormonal balance, focusing on the critical roles of negative and positive feedback loops in homeostasis. These principles are essential for understanding the complex interactions within the endocrine system and set the stage for more detailed discussions in subsequent chapters.

A solid grasp of these principles is crucial for both academic understanding and clinical applications, enabling the effective diagnosis and management of endocrine disorders. With this foundation, we are now prepared to delve into the specifics of hormonal assays and the physiology of various endocrine glands.

Case Studies

Case Study 1: Feedback Mechanisms in Hormonal Regulation

Patient Profile:

- Name: John Doe

- Age: 45 years

- Sex: Male

- Occupation: Office Worker

- Medical History: Mild hypertension, occasional headaches

- Family History: Father had diabetes type 2

Presentation:

John presents to his primary care physician with complaints of fatigue, unexplained weight gain, and feeling cold even in warm environments. He mentions that he has had difficulty concentrating at work and has been more forgetful lately. His wife has also noted that he appears more lethargic and has a low mood.

Physical Examination:

- Vital Signs: BP: 145/90 mmHg, HR: 60 bpm, Temp: 36.1°C

- General Appearance: Overweight, appears tired

- Thyroid Examination: Slightly enlarged thyroid gland

- Skin and Hair: Dry skin, thinning hair

Laboratory Tests:

- TSH (Thyroid-Stimulating Hormone): Elevated

- Free T4 (Thyroxine): Low

- Free T3 (Triiodothyronine): Low

Discussion:

John's presentation and laboratory findings suggest hypothyroidism, a condition where the thyroid gland is underactive. The elevated TSH levels indicate a feedback mechanism trying to stimulate the thyroid gland to produce more thyroid hormones (T3 and T4), which are crucial for metabolism and energy regulation.

Questions:

1. Explain the feedback mechanism involved in John's condition.

2. What is the role of TSH in thyroid hormone regulation?

3. Discuss the physiological effects of thyroid hormones on metabolism.

4. How does the negative feedback loop work in the context of thyroid hormone regulation?

Case Study 2: Hormonal Regulation in Stress Response

Patient Profile:

- Name: Jane Smith

- Age: 35 years

- Sex: Female

- Occupation: Lawyer

- Medical History: No significant past medical history

- Family History: Mother has hypertension

Presentation:

Jane presents with complaints of increased stress levels due to her demanding job. She reports difficulty sleeping, increased heart rate, and a sense of constant anxiety. She also mentions episodes of sudden sweating and palpitations.

Physical Examination:

- Vital Signs: BP: 130/85 mmHg, HR: 85 bpm, Temp: 36.8°C

- General Appearance: Appears anxious and restless

- Cardiovascular: No abnormalities detected

- Endocrine Examination: Normal

Laboratory Tests:

- Cortisol (Morning): Elevated

- ACTH (Adrenocorticotropic Hormone): Elevated

- Epinephrine and Norepinephrine: Elevated

Discussion:

Jane's symptoms and lab results suggest an overactive stress response, potentially indicative of chronic stress. The elevated cortisol and catecholamines (epinephrine and norepinephrine) are markers of the body's stress response, regulated by the hypothalamic-pituitary-adrenal (HPA) axis.

Questions:

1. Describe the role of the HPA axis in the stress response.

2. What are the physiological effects of cortisol and catecholamines during stress?

3. Explain the feedback mechanism involved in the regulation of cortisol.

4. How does chronic stress affect the endocrine system and overall health?

Practice Questions for Self-Assessment

Multiple Choice Questions

1. Which of the following is a primary function of hormones?

   a) Catalyze chemical reactions

   b) Transport oxygen in the blood

   c) Regulate physiological processes

   d) Provide structural support to cells

2. What type of hormone is derived from cholesterol?

   a) Peptide hormone

   b) Steroid hormone

   c) Amine hormone

   d) Glycoprotein hormone

3. Which of the following hormones is primarily involved in the regulation of blood calcium levels?

   a) Insulin

   b) Cortisol

   c) Parathyroid hormone (PTH)

   d) Thyroid hormone

4. The release of insulin from the pancreas in response to increased blood glucose levels is an example of:

   a) Positive feedback

   b) Negative feedback

   c) Feedforward control

   d) Hormonal antagonism

5. Which hormone is responsible for stimulating the production of milk in lactating women?

   a) Oxytocin

   b) Prolactin

   c) Estrogen

   d) Progesterone

Short Answer Questions

1. Define endocrinology and describe its significance in human physiology.

2. Explain the difference between autocrine, paracrine, and endocrine signaling.

3. Describe the mechanism of action for steroid hormones.

4. Discuss the role of feedback mechanisms in maintaining hormonal balance.

5. Explain how hormonal imbalances can lead to disease conditions, providing an example.

True or False Questions

1. TSH is produced by the thyroid gland. (True/False)

2. Hormones can only act on nearby target cells. (True/False)

3. The adrenal medulla secretes both cortisol and adrenaline. (True/False)

4. Insulin and glucagon have opposite effects on blood glucose levels. (True/False)

5. The hypothalamus directly secretes growth hormone. (True/False)

Answers

Case Study 1

1. Feedback Mechanism in John's Condition:

- John's elevated TSH and low thyroid hormone levels indicate a negative feedback mechanism. When thyroid hormone levels (T3 and T4) are low, the hypothalamus secretes thyrotropin-releasing hormone (TRH), which stimulates the pituitary to release TSH. TSH then stimulates the thyroid gland to produce and release T3 and T4. In hypothyroidism, the thyroid fails to produce sufficient hormones, leading to elevated TSH levels as the body attempts to compensate.

2. Role of TSH:

- TSH stimulates the thyroid gland to produce and release thyroid hormones (T3 and T4). It promotes thyroid cell growth and hormone synthesis, playing a crucial role in regulating metabolism, energy levels, and overall endocrine function.

3. Physiological Effects of Thyroid Hormones:

- Thyroid hormones increase the basal metabolic rate, enhance protein synthesis, stimulate carbohydrate and fat metabolism, and influence growth and development. They are critical for normal brain development and function, thermoregulation, and maintaining normal body weight.

4. Negative Feedback Loop in Thyroid Regulation:

- The negative feedback loop involves the hypothalamus, pituitary gland, and thyroid gland. Low thyroid hormone levels stimulate TRH release from the hypothalamus, which in turn stimulates TSH release from the pituitary. Elevated TSH levels stimulate the thyroid to produce more T3 and T4. As thyroid hormone levels rise, they inhibit TRH and TSH production, maintaining hormonal balance.

Case Study 2

1. Role of HPA Axis in Stress Response:

- The HPA axis is a central stress response system. Stress signals activate the hypothalamus to release corticotropin-releasing hormone (CRH), which stimulates the pituitary gland to secrete ACTH. ACTH then stimulates the adrenal cortex to produce cortisol. Cortisol helps mobilize energy, modulate immune responses, and maintain homeostasis during stress.

2. Physiological Effects of Cortisol and Catecholamines:

- Cortisol increases blood glucose levels, suppresses the immune system, and aids in metabolism. Catecholamines (epinephrine and norepinephrine) increase heart rate, blood pressure, and blood flow to muscles, preparing the body for a "fight or flight" response.

3. Feedback Mechanism in Cortisol Regulation:

- Cortisol exerts negative feedback on the hypothalamus and pituitary gland, inhibiting CRH and ACTH release. This feedback loop helps regulate cortisol levels, preventing excessive hormone secretion and maintaining balance.

4. Effects of Chronic Stress on the Endocrine System:

   - Chronic stress leads to prolonged HPA axis activation, resulting in elevated cortisol levels. This can cause immune suppression, increased blood pressure, altered glucose metabolism, and increased risk of mental health disorders such as anxiety and depression.

Multiple Choice Questions

1. c) Regulate physiological processes

2. b) Steroid hormone

3. c) Parathyroid hormone (PTH)

4. b) Negative feedback

5. b) Prolactin

Short Answer Questions

1. Endocrinology:

   - Endocrinology is the study of hormones, their receptors, and the intracellular signaling pathways they invoke. It is significant because hormones regulate critical physiological processes, including growth, metabolism, reproduction, and homeostasis.

2. Autocrine, Paracrine, Endocrine Signaling:

   - Autocrine signaling involves hormones acting on the same cell that secreted them. Paracrine signaling involves hormones acting on nearby cells. Endocrine signaling involves hormones being released into the bloodstream to act on distant target cells.

3. Mechanism of Action for Steroid Hormones:

   - Steroid hormones pass through cell membranes and bind to intracellular receptors. The hormone-receptor complex then enters the nucleus and regulates gene expression, leading to changes in protein synthesis and cell function.

4. Role of Feedback Mechanisms:

   - Feedback mechanisms maintain hormonal balance by regulating hormone levels. Negative feedback reduces the output of a hormone when its levels are high, while positive feedback amplifies hormone release in certain situations, ensuring stability and appropriate physiological responses.

5. Hormonal Imbalances and Disease:

- Hormonal imbalances can disrupt normal physiological processes, leading to diseases. For example, hyperthyroidism (excess thyroid hormone) can cause weight loss, increased heart rate, and nervousness, while hypothyroidism (deficient thyroid hormone) can lead to weight gain, fatigue, and depression.

True or False Questions

1. False

2. False

3. False

4. True

5. False

Bibliography

1. Williams, R. H., & Wilson, J. D. (2003). Williams Textbook of Endocrinology. Saunders.

   - This textbook provides an in-depth exploration of endocrine physiology, covering the classification, functions, and mechanisms of action of hormones, as well as feedback mechanisms. It is a foundational resource for understanding the principles of endocrinology.

2. Melmed, S., Polonsky, K. S., Larsen, P. R., & Kronenberg, H. M. (2011). Williams Textbook of Endocrinology (12th ed.). Elsevier.

   - This updated edition continues to serve as a comprehensive reference, delving into the latest research and developments in the field of endocrinology. It includes detailed chapters on hormone action and feedback regulation.

3. Guyton, A. C., & Hall, J. E. (2015). Textbook of Medical Physiology (13th ed.). Elsevier Saunders.

   - Guyton and Hall's textbook is a classic resource that provides clear explanations of physiological mechanisms, including those related to the endocrine system. It covers the fundamental principles and the intricate details of hormonal regulation.

4. Goodman, H. M. (2009). Basic Medical Endocrinology (4th ed.). Academic Press.

   - Goodman's textbook offers a concise yet thorough introduction to endocrinology, focusing on the basic principles and mechanisms of hormone action and regulation. It is well-suited for both beginners and advanced students.

5. Greenspan, F. S., & Gardner, D. G. (2004). Basic & Clinical Endocrinology (7th ed.). McGraw-Hill Medical.

   - This book bridges basic science and clinical practice, providing insights into the physiological principles of endocrinology and their application in clinical scenarios. It covers hormone classification, mechanisms of action, and feedback loops comprehensively.

6. Jameson, J. L., De Groot, L. J., & Weir, G. C. (2010). Endocrinology: Adult and Pediatric (6th ed.). Saunders.

   - This two-volume set provides extensive coverage of endocrine physiology, from basic concepts to clinical applications. It includes detailed discussions on the classification of hormones, their functions, and the regulatory mechanisms involved.

7. Kovacs, W. J., & Ojeda, S. R. (2012). Textbook of Endocrine Physiology (6th ed.). Oxford University Press.

   - This textbook offers a detailed examination of endocrine physiology, including the principles of hormone action and feedback mechanisms. It is a valuable resource for understanding the foundational aspects of endocrinology.

8. Nussey, S., & Whitehead, S. (2001). Endocrinology: An Integrated Approach. BIOS Scientific Publishers.

   - Nussey and Whitehead's book provides an integrated approach to endocrinology, combining basic science with clinical insights. It covers the principles of hormone action, regulation, and feedback in an accessible manner.

9. Strauss, J. F., & Barbieri, R. L. (2009). Yen and Jaffe's Reproductive Endocrinology: Physiology, Pathophysiology, and Clinical Management (6th ed.). Saunders.

   - Although focused on reproductive endocrinology, this book provides valuable insights into the general principles of endocrinology, including hormone classification, action, and feedback mechanisms.

10. Holt, R. I. G., Hanley, N. A., & Lamberts, S. W. J. (2010). Essential Endocrinology and Diabetes (6th ed.). Wiley-Blackwell.

    - This textbook offers a succinct yet comprehensive overview of endocrine physiology, with clear explanations of hormone classification, functions, and regulatory mechanisms. It is an excellent resource for both students and practitioners.

Chapter 2

Methods of Hormonal Assay

2.1 Overview of Hormonal Assays

Hormonal assays are essential laboratory techniques used to measure the concentration of hormones in biological samples, such as blood, urine, or saliva. These assays provide valuable information about hormone levels, which is crucial for diagnosing endocrine disorders, monitoring treatment efficacy, and conducting research in endocrinology. Various methods have been developed for hormonal assays, each with its advantages and limitations.

Types of Hormonal Assays:

Hormonal assays encompass a variety of techniques designed to measure the concentration of hormones in biological samples accurately. Each method has its unique principles, advantages, and limitations.

1. Immunoassay Techniques:

- Enzyme-Linked Immunosorbent Assay (ELISA): ELISA is a widely used immunoassay technique in which an antigen of interest, typically a hormone, is immobilized on a solid surface (e.g., microplate wells). Enzyme-labeled antibodies specific to the target hormone are added, and after incubation and washing steps, a substrate solution is added. The enzyme catalyzes a colorimetric or fluorescent reaction, and the intensity of the signal is proportional to the hormone concentration in the sample. ELISA offers high sensitivity, specificity, and flexibility in assay design, making it suitable for a wide range of applications, including clinical diagnostics, drug discovery, and research.

- Radioimmunoassay (RIA): RIA is a sensitive technique used to measure hormone concentrations by utilizing the competitive binding of a radioactive-labeled hormone and an unlabeled hormone in the sample to specific antibodies. After incubation, separation of bound and unbound fractions is performed, and the radioactivity of the bound fraction is measured using a scintillation counter. The amount of radioactive signal is inversely proportional to the concentration of unlabeled hormone in the sample. RIA offers high sensitivity and specificity but has declined in popularity due to safety concerns associated with radioactive materials and regulatory restrictions.

- Chemiluminescent Immunoassay (CLIA): CLIA utilizes chemiluminescent compounds (e.g., acridinium esters) as labels for antibodies to detect hormone-antibody complexes. Upon binding, the chemiluminescent reaction is triggered, producing light emission proportional to the hormone concentration. CLIA offers advantages such as enhanced sensitivity, wider dynamic range, and automation capabilities compared to traditional immunoassays. It is commonly used in clinical laboratories for high-throughput hormone testing, particularly in automated platforms.

2. Mass Spectrometry:

- Liquid Chromatography-Tandem Mass Spectrometry (LC-MS/MS): LC-MS/MS is a highly sensitive and specific technique used for quantifying hormones based on their mass-to-charge ratio. In LC-MS/MS, biological samples are first separated using liquid chromatography to isolate the target hormone from other molecules. The separated analytes are then ionized and fragmented in the mass spectrometer, and the resulting mass spectra are analyzed to determine the abundance of the hormone. LC-MS/MS offers multiplexing capabilities, allowing simultaneous measurement of multiple hormones in a single sample with high accuracy and precision. It is particularly suitable for measuring steroid hormones and peptides with complex molecular structures and has become increasingly popular in clinical and research laboratories for hormone analysis.

3. Other Techniques:

- Bioassays: Bioassays involve the use of living cells, tissues, or organisms to measure hormone activity or biological effects. These assays assess the physiological response elicited by the hormone and can provide valuable information about hormone potency, bioavailability, and receptor activation. Although less commonly used than immunoassays or mass spectrometry, bioassays are employed for specific hormones or research purposes, particularly when assessing hormone bioactivity.

- Receptor Binding Assays: Receptor binding assays measure the binding affinity and kinetics of hormones to their specific receptors. These assays typically involve the use of radiolabeled ligands to quantify receptor-ligand interactions and assess hormone potency and activity. Receptor binding assays provide insights into the mechanisms of hormone action and receptor pharmacology and are valuable tools in drug development and research.

- Molecular Assays (e.g., PCR): Molecular assays such as polymerase chain reaction (PCR) are used to quantify gene expression levels of hormone-related genes or detect specific genetic mutations associated with endocrine disorders. These assays amplify and detect nucleic acid sequences corresponding to target genes, providing information about gene expression patterns, mutations, and polymorphisms relevant to endocrine function and pathology.

Advantages of Hormonal Assays:

Hormonal assays serve as indispensable tools in both clinical practice and research, offering a multitude of advantages that contribute to their widespread adoption and utility. Let's delve into these advantages in finer detail:

1. High Sensitivity:

- Hormonal assays boast exceptional sensitivity, enabling the detection and quantification of hormones even at minute concentrations within biological samples. This sensitivity allows for the early detection of endocrine disorders and facilitates the monitoring of subtle changes in hormone levels over time.

2. Specificity:

- One of the hallmark features of hormonal assays is their high specificity. These assays accurately measure the concentration of a particular hormone without interference from other molecules present in the sample. Utilizing specific antibodies or molecular probes tailored to the hormone of interest ensures precise and reliable results.

3. Quantitative Precision:

- Hormonal assays provide quantitative data on hormone levels, allowing for precise measurement and comparison across individuals or experimental conditions. This quantitative precision is invaluable in clinical settings for monitoring treatment efficacy, establishing reference ranges, and discerning pathological states from normal physiology.

4. Clinical Relevance:

- Hormonal assays have immense clinical relevance, serving as pivotal diagnostic tools for identifying endocrine disorders, guiding treatment decisions, and monitoring patient health. By accurately assessing hormone levels, these assays empower healthcare professionals to deliver personalized and targeted interventions.

5. Versatility and Adaptability:

- Hormonal assays exhibit remarkable versatility and can be adapted to measure a diverse array of hormones and biomarkers across various sample types, including blood, urine, saliva, and tissue specimens. This adaptability enables researchers and clinicians to explore a wide spectrum of endocrine functions and pathologies.

6. Automation and Throughput:

- Many hormonal assays are amenable to automation, facilitating high-throughput analysis of large sample volumes. Automated platforms enhance assay efficiency, minimize manual errors, and expedite sample processing, making them indispensable tools for clinical laboratories handling extensive sample queues.

7. Facilitation of Research Endeavors:

- Hormonal assays play a pivotal role in advancing scientific knowledge and understanding in the field of endocrinology. By enabling the investigation of hormone regulation, physiological responses, and disease mechanisms, these assays drive innovation and inform the development of novel therapeutic strategies.

8. Long-Term Stability and Reliability:

- Hormonal assays often employ stable reagents and detection methodologies, ensuring the long-term stability and reproducibility of results. This reliability extends to sample storage, allowing for the preservation of samples over extended periods without compromising assay accuracy.

Limitations and Challenges:

1. Variability in Sample Matrix: Biological samples, such as blood or urine, can contain interfering substances that affect assay accuracy and reproducibility. Variations in sample matrix composition between individuals or over time can introduce variability in hormone measurements.

2. Standardization: The lack of standardized protocols, reference materials, and quality control measures poses challenges for ensuring consistency and comparability between different assay platforms and laboratories. Variations in assay procedures and reagents can lead to discrepancies in hormone measurements.

3. Cost and Time: Some hormonal assays may be expensive and time-consuming, requiring specialized equipment and reagents. High costs associated with assay kits, instrumentation, and personnel training can limit the accessibility and scalability of hormonal testing, particularly in resource-limited settings.

4. Interference: Endogenous substances present in biological samples, such as lipids, proteins, or metabolites, as well as medications or dietary supplements, can interfere with hormone measurements. Careful sample preparation and validation are necessary to minimize interference and ensure the accuracy of hormone assays.

5. Dynamic Range and Sensitivity: Hormonal assays must be able to detect hormones over a wide range of concentrations, from picograms to nanograms per milliliter, to accommodate physiological variations and disease states. Achieving optimal sensitivity without sacrificing specificity can be challenging, particularly for hormones present at low levels.

6. Cross-reactivity: Immunoassays may exhibit cross-reactivity with structurally similar molecules, leading to false-positive or false-negative results. Selecting antibodies with high specificity and minimizing nonspecific binding are critical for minimizing cross-reactivity in hormonal assays.

7. Sample Storage and Stability: Proper sample handling, storage, and transportation are essential for preserving hormone stability and preventing degradation. Factors such as temperature fluctuations, pH changes, and freeze-thaw cycles can affect hormone integrity and compromise assay reliability.

8. Biological Variability: Biological factors, such as circadian rhythms, age, sex, hormonal fluctuations, and underlying medical conditions, can influence hormone levels and introduce variability in assay results. Standardizing sampling protocols and accounting for biological variability are necessary for accurate interpretation of hormone measurements.

Future Directions in Hormonal Assays:

1. Technological Advances: Continued research and development efforts are expected to lead to the refinement and optimization of hormonal assay technologies. This includes the exploration of novel detection methods, such as nanotechnology-based sensors, microfluidic devices, and advanced imaging techniques, to improve assay sensitivity, specificity, and speed.

2. Standardization Efforts: Collaborative initiatives among researchers, clinicians, and regulatory agencies aim to establish standardized protocols, reference materials, and quality control measures for hormonal assays. This will facilitate comparability between different laboratories and assay platforms, ensuring reliable and reproducible results.

3. Point-of-Care Testing (POCT): The development of miniaturized assay platforms and portable devices enables decentralized testing at the point of care, allowing for rapid and convenient hormone measurement in clinical settings, remote areas, and resource-limited environments. POCT for hormones holds great potential for timely diagnosis, monitoring, and management of endocrine disorders.

4. Multiplex Assays: Multiplexed immunoassays and mass spectrometry-based platforms enable the simultaneous measurement of multiple hormones in a single sample, offering a comprehensive assessment of endocrine function. Multiplex assays improve efficiency, reduce sample volume requirements, and provide valuable insights into hormone interactions and regulatory networks.

5. Integration with Omics Technologies: Integration of hormonal assays with omics technologies, such as genomics, transcriptomics, proteomics, and metabolomics, offers a holistic approach to studying endocrine function and disease. This multi-omics approach allows for the identification of biomarkers, elucidation of disease mechanisms, and personalized treatment strategies tailored to individual hormonal profiles.

6. Biosensors and Wearable Devices: Advancements in biosensor technology enable real-time monitoring of hormone levels through wearable devices, smart textiles, and implantable sensors. Continuous monitoring of hormones provides valuable longitudinal data, allowing for early detection of abnormalities, optimization of treatment regimens, and personalized interventions for hormone-related conditions.

7. Artificial Intelligence (AI) and Machine Learning: Integration of AI algorithms and machine learning models with hormonal assay data facilitates data analysis, pattern recognition, and predictive modeling for disease diagnosis, prognosis, and treatment optimization. AI-driven approaches enhance the interpretation of complex hormonal data, leading to more precise and personalized healthcare interventions.

8. Biomedical Engineering Innovations: Collaborations between biomedical engineers, chemists, and biologists are driving innovations in assay design, microfluidics, biomaterials, and lab-on-a-chip technologies for hormonal measurement. These interdisciplinary efforts aim to address current limitations in assay performance, scalability, and accessibility, paving the way for next-generation hormonal assays with enhanced capabilities.

2.2 Immunoassay Techniques

Immunoassay techniques are widely employed for measuring hormone levels due to their high sensitivity, specificity, and versatility. These assays rely on the selective binding between antigens (hormones) and antibodies, enabling the detection and quantification of target hormones in biological samples. Several immunoassay techniques are commonly used in endocrinology, including:

Enzyme-Linked Immunosorbent Assay (ELISA)

Enzyme-Linked Immunosorbent Assay (ELISA) is a sensitive and versatile laboratory technique used to detect and quantify the presence of a specific substance, such as a hormone, antigen, antibody, or protein, in a biological sample. ELISA is widely employed in various fields, including clinical diagnostics, biomedical research, pharmaceutical development, and food safety testing, due to its high sensitivity, specificity, and ease of automation.

Principle of ELISA:

The principle of ELISA is based on the specific binding between an antigen (the substance to be detected) and an antibody (a protein that recognizes and binds to the antigen) immobilized on a solid support surface, typically a microplate. ELISA can be performed in different formats, including direct, indirect, sandwich, and competitive assays, depending on the specific application and the target molecule.

Key Steps of ELISA:

1. Coating: The wells of a microplate are coated with a capture antibody that specifically binds to the target antigen.

2. Blocking: Unoccupied binding sites on the microplate surface are blocked with a blocking agent, such as bovine serum albumin (BSA) or casein, to prevent nonspecific binding of other proteins or substances in the sample.

3. Sample Incubation: The sample containing the antigen of interest is added to the microplate wells and allowed to incubate. During this incubation period, the antigen binds to the immobilized capture antibody, forming an antigen-antibody complex.

4. Washing: After the incubation, the microplate wells are washed multiple times with a wash buffer to remove unbound substances and reduce background noise.

5. Detection: A secondary antibody, conjugated to an enzyme (e.g., horseradish peroxidase or alkaline phosphatase), is added to the wells. This secondary antibody specifically binds to the antigen-antibody complex formed in the previous step.

6. Substrate Addition: A substrate specific to the enzyme is added to the wells. The enzyme catalyzes a reaction with the substrate, resulting in the production of a detectable signal, typically a color change or fluorescent emission.

7. Signal Measurement: The intensity of the generated signal is proportional to the amount of antigen present in the sample. The signal is measured using a spectrophotometer or a fluorescence reader, and the concentration of the antigen in the sample is determined based on a standard curve generated using known concentrations of the antigen.

Types of ELISA:

- Direct ELISA: Involves direct binding of a labeled detection antibody to the captured antigen.

- Indirect ELISA: Utilizes a secondary antibody labeled with an enzyme to detect the bound antigen-antibody complex.

- Sandwich ELISA: Uses two antibodies (capture and detection) to sandwich the antigen, increasing specificity and sensitivity.

- Competitive ELISA: Involves competition between labeled and unlabeled antigens for binding to a limited number of antibodies, allowing quantification based on inhibition of signal.

Applications of ELISA:

ELISA has a wide range of applications in various fields, including:

- Clinical diagnostics for detecting hormones, antibodies, and biomarkers associated with diseases.

- Pharmaceutical research and development for drug screening and monitoring.

- Immunology research for studying immune responses and antibody detection.

- Food safety testing for detecting allergens and contaminants.

Radioimmunoassay (RIA)

Radioimmunoassay (RIA) is a highly sensitive laboratory technique used to measure the concentration of specific substances, such as hormones, drugs, or proteins, in biological samples. RIA utilizes the competitive binding principle between a radioactive-labeled (tracer) antigen and an unlabeled antigen for a limited number of specific antibodies. This technique was developed in the late 1950s by Dr. Rosalyn Sussman Yalow and Dr. Solomon A. Berson and has since become a valuable tool in clinical diagnostics, pharmaceutical research, and biomedical science.

Principle of RIA:

The principle of RIA is based on the competitive binding between a known amount of radioactive-labeled antigen (tracer) and an unlabeled antigen present in the sample for a limited number of specific antibodies. The steps involved in RIA are as follows:

1. Preparation of Tracer: A known quantity of the antigen of interest is labeled with a radioactive isotope, such as iodine-125 (^{125}I) or tritium (^{3}H), to produce the radioactive-labeled antigen (tracer). The tracer should retain the biological activity of the unlabeled antigen.

2. Antibody Coating: Antibodies specific to the antigen are immobilized onto a solid-phase support, such as a plastic tube or microplate, to capture the antigen-antibody complex.

3. Sample Incubation: The sample containing the unlabeled antigen is added to the solid-phase support containing the immobilized antibodies. Simultaneously, a known amount of radioactive-labeled antigen (tracer) is added to the sample.

4. Competitive Binding: Both the unlabeled antigen in the sample and the radioactive-labeled antigen (tracer) compete for binding to the limited number of specific antibodies. The proportion of bound tracer and unlabeled antigen depends on their respective concentrations in the sample.

5. Separation of Bound and Free Fractions: After an incubation period, the unbound (free) and bound fractions are separated. This can be achieved by techniques such as precipitation, centrifugation, or filtration.

6. Radioactivity Measurement: The radioactivity of either the bound or free fraction is measured using a gamma counter. The amount of radioactivity detected is inversely proportional to the concentration of unlabeled antigen in the sample.

7. Calculation of Antigen Concentration: The concentration of the unlabeled antigen in the sample is determined by comparing the measured radioactivity to a standard curve generated using known concentrations of the antigen.

Advantages of RIA:

- High Sensitivity: RIA can detect antigens at very low concentrations, often in the picomolar or femtomolar range.

- High Specificity: RIA relies on the specific binding between antigens and antibodies, ensuring accurate detection of target molecules.

- Wide Dynamic Range: RIA can measure a wide range of antigen concentrations without the need for sample dilution.

Applications of RIA:

RIA has numerous applications in various fields, including:

- Clinical Diagnostics: Measurement of hormones, drugs, and tumor markers in patient samples.

- Pharmaceutical Research: Pharmacokinetic studies, drug metabolism, and receptor binding assays.

- Biomedical Research: Investigation of hormone regulation, immune responses, and protein-protein interactions.

Chemiluminescent Immunoassay (CLIA)

Chemiluminescent Immunoassay (CLIA) is a highly sensitive immunoassay technique used for the quantitative measurement of hormones, antibodies, proteins, and other biomolecules in biological samples. CLIA offers several advantages, including high sensitivity, wide dynamic range, and rapid assay kinetics, making it an attractive alternative to traditional immunoassay methods such as ELISA.

Principle:

The principle of CLIA is based on the specific binding between an antigen (hormone) and an antibody, which is labeled with a chemiluminescent compound. The assay involves several key steps:

1. Coating: The solid-phase surface, typically a microplate, is coated with capture antibodies that specifically bind to the target hormone.

2. Sample Incubation: The sample containing the hormone of interest is added to the microplate wells and allowed to incubate. During this incubation, the hormone binds to the immobilized capture antibodies, forming a hormone-antibody complex.

3. Washing: After the incubation period, the microplate wells are washed to remove unbound substances and reduce background noise.

4. Detection: A detection antibody labeled with a chemiluminescent compound (e.g., acridinium ester or luminol) is added to the wells. This detection antibody specifically binds to the hormone-antibody complex, forming a sandwich-like structure.

5. Triggering Reaction: Addition of a triggering reagent, such as hydrogen peroxide, initiates a chemiluminescent reaction with the labeled antibody. This reaction produces light emission proportional to the concentration of the hormone in the sample.

6. Signal Measurement: The emitted light is measured using a luminometer, and the intensity of the light emission is quantified. The signal intensity is proportional to the concentration of the hormone in the sample.

Advantages of CLIA:

- High Sensitivity: CLIA offers exceptional sensitivity, allowing detection of hormones at low concentrations, even in complex biological matrices.

- Wide Dynamic Range: CLIA has a wide dynamic range, enabling accurate measurement of hormone levels across a broad concentration range.

- Rapid Assay Kinetics: CLIA assays typically have rapid assay kinetics, allowing for faster turnaround times and higher throughput compared to traditional immunoassays.

- Reduced Background Noise: CLIA assays often exhibit lower background noise due to the absence of light scatter, resulting in improved signal-to-noise ratios and assay precision.

Applications:

CLIA has diverse applications in clinical diagnostics, research, and drug development, including:

- Measurement of hormone levels for diagnosing endocrine disorders and monitoring treatment efficacy.

- Detection of biomarkers associated with various diseases, including cancer, infectious diseases, and autoimmune disorders.

- Drug screening and pharmacokinetic studies in pharmaceutical research.

- Immunological assays for studying immune responses and antibody detection.

2.5 Mass Spectrometry

Mass spectrometry (MS) is a powerful analytical technique used for quantifying hormones and other biomolecules based on their mass-to-charge ratio (m/z). Mass spectrometry offers several advantages for hormonal assays, including high sensitivity, specificity, and the ability to analyze multiple analytes simultaneously.

Principles of Mass Spectrometry:

Mass spectrometry operates on the principle of ionization, separation, and detection of ions based on their mass-to-charge ratio. The sample is first ionized, typically using techniques such as electrospray ionization (ESI) or atmospheric pressure chemical ionization (APCI), generating ions that are then separated based on their mass-to-charge ratio in the mass analyzer. Finally, the ions are detected, and their abundance is quantified, allowing the determination of the concentration of analytes present in the sample.

Liquid Chromatography-Tandem Mass Spectrometry (LC-MS/MS):

Liquid chromatography-tandem mass spectrometry (LC-MS/MS) is a widely used technique for hormonal assays, particularly for measuring steroid hormones and peptide hormones. In LC-MS/MS, the sample is first separated by liquid chromatography based on its chemical properties, followed by ionization and detection by mass spectrometry. LC-MS/MS offers excellent sensitivity and specificity, allowing for accurate quantification of hormones even at low concentrations. It also enables multiplexed analysis of multiple analytes in a single run, making it a valuable tool for comprehensive endocrine profiling.

Advantages of Mass Spectrometry in Hormonal Assays:

1. High Sensitivity: Mass spectrometry offers high sensitivity, allowing for the detection of hormones at low concentrations, which is particularly important for measuring hormones present in trace amounts in biological samples.

2. Specificity: Mass spectrometry provides high specificity, enabling accurate identification and quantification of hormones even in complex biological matrices containing interfering substances.

3. Multiplexing: Mass spectrometry allows for the simultaneous analysis of multiple analytes in a single run, providing comprehensive information about the endocrine profile of an individual.

4. Accuracy and Precision: Mass spectrometry-based assays offer excellent accuracy and precision, making them suitable for clinical diagnostics and research applications.

5. Versatility: Mass spectrometry can be applied to measure a wide range of hormones, including steroids, peptides, and small molecules, making it a versatile tool for endocrine research and diagnostics.

Challenges and Considerations:

While mass spectrometry offers numerous advantages for hormonal assays, it also presents some challenges, including the need for specialized instrumentation, technical expertise, and optimization of assay parameters. Sample preparation and matrix effects can also influence assay performance and require careful consideration. Despite these challenges, mass spectrometry remains a valuable technique for advancing our understanding of endocrine physiology and diagnosing endocrine disorders.

2.6 Conclusion

This chapter provided a comprehensive overview of the methods utilized in measuring hormone levels, a critical aspect of both research and clinical practice in endocrine physiology. We introduced the significance of hormonal assays in understanding endocrine function and diagnosing related disorders.

Various techniques were explored, including radioimmunoassay (RIA), enzyme-linked immunosorbent assay (ELISA), and other advanced methodologies, each offering distinct advantages and considerations. Understanding how to interpret assay results involves careful consideration of assay parameters and clinical context.

Mastering these techniques enables researchers and clinicians to accurately assess hormone levels, contributing to both patient care and advancements in endocrine research. As we proceed, we will apply these methods to explore the physiology of specific endocrine glands, further enriching our understanding of this intricate field.

Case Studies

Case Study 1: Diagnosing Cushing's Syndrome

Patient Profile:

- Name: Emily Johnson

- Age: 50 years

- Sex: Female

- Occupation: Teacher

- Medical History: Hypertension, osteoporosis

- Family History: No significant history

Presentation:

Emily visits her endocrinologist with complaints of weight gain, particularly around her abdomen and face, increased bruising, and muscle weakness. She also reports feeling fatigued and having mood swings.

Physical Examination:

- Vital Signs: BP: 150/95 mmHg, HR: 80 bpm, Temp: 37.0°C

- General Appearance: Central obesity, moon face, and buffalo hump

- Skin Examination: Purple striae on the abdomen, easy bruising

Laboratory Tests:

- Initial Blood Tests: Elevated blood glucose, low potassium

- 24-hour Urinary Free Cortisol: Elevated

- Midnight Serum Cortisol: Elevated

- Low-dose Dexamethasone Suppression Test: No suppression of cortisol

Discussion:

Emily's symptoms and laboratory findings are indicative of Cushing's syndrome, a condition characterized by excessive cortisol production. The hormonal assays used, including the 24-hour urinary free cortisol and the dexamethasone suppression test, help confirm the diagnosis by demonstrating abnormal cortisol regulation.

Questions:

1. Describe the principles behind the 24-hour urinary free cortisol test and its significance.

2. Explain the rationale for using the low-dose dexamethasone suppression test in diagnosing Cushing's syndrome.

3. What are the potential pitfalls and limitations of these hormonal assays?

4. Discuss the role of midnight serum cortisol measurement in the assessment of Cushing's syndrome.

Case Study 2: Assessing Thyroid Function

Patient Profile:

- Name: Mark Thompson

- Age: 35 years

- Sex: Male

- Occupation: IT Specialist

- Medical History: Mild asthma

- Family History: Mother had hypothyroidism

Presentation:

Mark presents with symptoms of fatigue, weight gain, and constipation. He reports feeling unusually cold and has noticed swelling in his neck.

Physical Examination:

- Vital Signs: BP: 120/80 mmHg, HR: 65 bpm, Temp: 36.5°C

- Thyroid Examination: Palpable goiter

- Skin Examination: Dry skin, coarse hair

Laboratory Tests:

- TSH (Thyroid-Stimulating Hormone): Elevated

- Free T4 (Thyroxine): Low

- Anti-thyroid Antibodies: Positive for anti-TPO antibodies

Discussion:

Mark's clinical presentation and laboratory results suggest primary hypothyroidism, likely due to Hashimoto's thyroiditis. The elevated TSH and low free T4 levels indicate a primary thyroid dysfunction, while the presence of anti-thyroid antibodies confirms an autoimmune etiology.

Questions:

1. Discuss the significance of measuring TSH and free T4 in diagnosing thyroid disorders.

2. Explain the importance of anti-thyroid antibody testing in the context of hypothyroidism.

3. Describe the method of performing a TSH assay.

4. What are the advantages and limitations of using serum TSH as a screening test for thyroid dysfunction?

Practice Questions for Self-Assessment

Multiple Choice Questions

1. Which of the following is a commonly used technique for measuring hormone levels in the blood?

   a) Western blot

   b) Polymerase chain reaction (PCR)

   c) Enzyme-linked immunosorbent assay (ELISA)

   d) Southern blot

2. The principle of radioimmunoassay (RIA) involves:

a) Competitive binding of radio-labeled and non-radio-labeled antigens

b) Detection of nucleic acids

c) Separation of proteins by size

d) Measurement of enzyme activity

3. Which hormone is typically measured using a 24-hour urine collection?

a) Insulin

b) Cortisol

c) TSH

d) Estrogen

4. The dexamethasone suppression test is used to assess the function of the:

a) Thyroid gland

b) Adrenal cortex

c) Pituitary gland

d) Pancreas

5. An elevated TSH level with a low free T4 suggests:

a) Primary hyperthyroidism

b) Secondary hypothyroidism

c) Primary hypothyroidism

d) Euthyroid sick syndrome

Short Answer Questions

1. Describe the principle of enzyme-linked immunosorbent assay (ELISA).

2. Explain how radioimmunoassay (RIA) is used to measure hormone levels.

3. Discuss the clinical utility of 24-hour urinary hormone assays.

4. Describe the steps involved in performing a low-dose dexamethasone suppression test.

5. Explain how the presence of anti-thyroid antibodies can influence the diagnosis and management of thyroid disorders.

True or False Questions

1. ELISA is a technique used to measure hormone levels by detecting specific antibodies. (True/False)

2. The 24-hour urinary free cortisol test is used to diagnose thyroid disorders. (True/False)

3. Radioimmunoassay (RIA) requires the use of radio-labeled hormones. (True/False)

4. High levels of TSH with high levels of free T4 indicate primary hypothyroidism. (True/False)

5. The dexamethasone suppression test helps diagnose disorders related to cortisol production. (True/False)

Answers

Case Study 1

1. Principles Behind 24-hour Urinary Free Cortisol Test:

- This test measures the amount of cortisol excreted in the urine over 24 hours, providing an integrated measure of cortisol production. It is significant as it reflects the body's cortisol production and is used to diagnose conditions of cortisol excess, such as Cushing's syndrome.

2. Rationale for Low-dose Dexamethasone Suppression Test:

- The low-dose dexamethasone suppression test assesses the feedback regulation of the hypothalamic-pituitary-adrenal (HPA) axis. In normal individuals, dexamethasone suppresses cortisol production. Lack of suppression in patients suggests hypercortisolism, as seen in Cushing's syndrome.

3. Pitfalls and Limitations of Hormonal Assays:

- Potential pitfalls include variability in urine collection for 24-hour tests, cross-reactivity in immunoassays, and false positives/negatives. The dexamethasone suppression test may be affected by patient compliance, timing of sample collection, and concurrent medications.

4. Role of Midnight Serum Cortisol Measurement:

- Measuring cortisol levels at midnight helps identify abnormal diurnal variation in cortisol secretion, which is often elevated in patients with Cushing's syndrome. This time point is chosen because cortisol levels should be low at night in healthy individuals.

Case Study 2

1. Significance of Measuring TSH and Free T4:

- TSH and free T4 levels are critical for diagnosing thyroid disorders. Elevated TSH with low free T4 suggests primary hypothyroidism, indicating a thyroid gland issue. Low TSH with low free T4 suggests central hypothyroidism, indicating a pituitary or hypothalamic issue.

2. Importance of Anti-thyroid Antibody Testing:

- Anti-thyroid antibodies, such as anti-TPO antibodies, are markers of autoimmune thyroid disease. Their presence in hypothyroid patients suggests Hashimoto's thyroiditis, guiding treatment and management.

3. Method of Performing a TSH Assay:

- A TSH assay is typically performed using immunoassay techniques like ELISA. The patient's blood sample is mixed with antibodies specific to TSH, which bind to the hormone and generate a measurable signal, indicating the TSH concentration.

4. Advantages and Limitations of Serum TSH:

- Advantages: Sensitive marker for thyroid function, helps differentiate between primary and secondary thyroid disorders, non-invasive, and widely available.

- Limitations: TSH levels can be influenced by non-thyroidal illness, medications, and time of day; may not reflect acute changes in thyroid status.

Multiple Choice Questions

1. c) Enzyme-linked immunosorbent assay (ELISA)

2. a) Competitive binding of radio-labeled and non-radio-labeled antigens

3. b) Cortisol

4. b) Adrenal cortex

5. c) Primary hypothyroidism

Short Answer Questions

1. Principle of ELISA:

- ELISA is a biochemical technique used to detect and quantify substances, usually antigens or antibodies. It relies on antigen-antibody interactions, where an enzyme-linked antibody binds to the target antigen. A substrate is then added, which the enzyme converts to a detectable signal, often a color change, indicating the presence and quantity of the antigen.

2. Radioimmunoassay (RIA):

- RIA measures hormone levels by using radio-labeled hormones that compete with the hormone in the patient's sample to bind to specific antibodies. The bound and free hormones are separated, and the radioactivity of the bound fraction is measured, which is inversely proportional to the hormone concentration in the sample.

3. Clinical Utility of 24-hour Urinary Hormone Assays:

- These assays provide a comprehensive measure of hormone production over a day, useful for diagnosing conditions with diurnal variation or intermittent secretion. They are commonly used for assessing cortisol levels in suspected Cushing's syndrome or adrenal insufficiency.

4. Low-dose Dexamethasone Suppression Test:

- The patient takes dexamethasone, a synthetic glucocorticoid, usually at a dose of 1 mg at 11 PM. Blood samples are taken the next morning to measure cortisol levels. Normal suppression of cortisol indicates a functional HPA axis, while lack of suppression suggests hypercortisolism.

5. Anti-thyroid Antibodies:

- The presence of anti-thyroid antibodies suggests an autoimmune thyroid disorder, such as Hashimoto's thyroiditis or Graves' disease. These antibodies can damage thyroid tissue, leading to hypothyroidism or hyperthyroidism, and guide the diagnosis and management plan.

True or False Questions

1. False

2. False

3. True

4. False

5. True

Bibliography

1. Burtis, C. A., & Bruns, D. E. (2012). Tietz fundamentals of clinical chemistry and molecular diagnostics (7th ed.). Elsevier Saunders.

   - This textbook provides an extensive overview of clinical chemistry techniques, including hormonal assays such as radioimmunoassay and enzyme-linked immunosorbent assay (ELISA).

2. Melmed, S., Polonsky, K. S., Larsen, P. R., & Kronenberg, H. M. (Eds.). (2016). Williams textbook of endocrinology (13th ed.). Elsevier.

   - Chapter 7, "Assessment of Endocrine Function", discusses various methods for measuring hormone levels, offering insights into the principles and applications of different assays.

3. Wu, A. H. B., & Tietz, N. W. (Eds.). (2011). Tietz clinical guide to laboratory tests (4th ed.). Saunders.

   - This guide includes detailed protocols and interpretations of laboratory tests, including hormonal assays, useful for understanding the practical aspects of hormone measurement techniques.

4. Kricka, L. J. (2006). Principles and practice of immunoassay (2nd ed.). Academic Press.

   - This book focuses on immunoassay principles, covering radioimmunoassay and newer technologies like ELISA, providing in-depth information on assay methodologies.

5. Lepage, N., & Dufour, D. R. (2001). Clinical chemistry and laboratory medicine: Methods and interpretations. Lippincott Williams & Wilkins.

   - Chapter 10, "Immunochemical Techniques", discusses the principles and applications of immunoassays, including their relevance in clinical endocrinology.

Chapter 3

Physiology of the Endocrine Hypothalamus

The hypothalamus produces a variety of releasing and inhibiting hormones that regulate the secretion of pituitary hormones. These hypothalamic hormones are crucial for coordinating the activity of the pituitary gland and, consequently, the function of peripheral endocrine organs. Here, we explore the key hypothalamic hormones and their regulatory mechanisms:

3.1 Anatomy and Function of the Hypothalamus

Anatomy of the Hypothalamus

The hypothalamus, a vital structure located below the thalamus and above the brainstem, is a small but incredibly important part of the brain. Its anatomy is intricate, consisting of several nuclei and pathways that contribute to its diverse functions.

Location:

- Situated in the diencephalon, at the base of the brain.

- Forms the floor and part of the lateral walls of the third ventricle, a fluid-filled cavity within the brain.

Structural Components:

Nuclei: The hypothalamus contains numerous nuclei, each with specific functions. Some of the key nuclei include:

  - Paraventricular nucleus: Involved in regulating hormone secretion from the pituitary gland and autonomic functions.

  - Supraoptic nucleus: Produces vasopressin (antidiuretic hormone) and oxytocin, which are stored and released by the posterior pituitary gland.

  - Arcuate nucleus: Regulates appetite and energy balance, containing neurons sensitive to hunger and satiety signals.

  - Ventromedial nucleus: Also involved in appetite regulation, particularly in response to satiety signals.

  - Suprachiasmatic nucleus: Controls circadian rhythms, serving as the body's internal clock.

Connections:

The hypothalamus has extensive connections with other brain regions and peripheral organs, allowing it to integrate sensory input and coordinate appropriate responses. Key connections include:

- Pituitary gland: The hypothalamus communicates with the pituitary gland (both anterior and posterior lobes) via neural and vascular pathways, regulating hormone secretion.

- Limbic system: Receives input from regions involved in emotion and behavior, influencing autonomic and endocrine responses to stress and emotional stimuli.

- Brainstem: Receives input from and sends projections to the brainstem, coordinating autonomic functions such as heart rate, blood pressure, and respiration.

- Higher brain centers: Integrates signals from cortical and subcortical regions involved in cognition, perception, and consciousness, modulating hypothalamic functions.

Vascular Supply:

- The hypothalamus receives its blood supply from branches of the anterior and posterior cerebral arteries, as well as the circle of Willis, ensuring adequate oxygen and nutrient delivery to this metabolically active region.

Functional Organization:

- The hypothalamus is functionally organized into distinct nuclei and pathways, each contributing to specific physiological processes such as hormone secretion, autonomic control, temperature regulation, appetite, thirst, and circadian rhythms.

Functions of the Hypothalamus:

1. Regulation of Hormone Secretion: The hypothalamus produces releasing and inhibiting hormones that control the secretion of pituitary hormones involved in growth, metabolism, reproduction, and stress response. This regulation occurs through the hypothalamo-pituitary axis, which integrates hormonal signals and feedback mechanisms to maintain hormonal balance.

2. Autonomic Nervous System Control: The hypothalamus regulates the autonomic nervous system, which controls involuntary bodily functions such as heart rate, blood pressure, digestion, and respiratory rate. It modulates sympathetic and parasympathetic output in response to changes in internal and external stimuli, helping to maintain physiological equilibrium.

3. Temperature Regulation: Acting as the body's thermostat, the hypothalamus monitors core body temperature and orchestrates physiological responses to maintain homeostasis. These responses include adjustments in peripheral blood flow, sweat production, and shivering, ensuring that body temperature remains within a narrow range despite fluctuations in environmental temperature.

4. Hunger and Satiety: Specific nuclei within the hypothalamus regulate appetite and energy balance by integrating hormonal, neural, and metabolic signals. This regulation helps modulate feeding behavior, energy expenditure, and adipose tissue metabolism to ensure adequate nutrient intake and energy balance.

5. Thirst and Fluid Balance: The hypothalamus monitors osmotic pressure and sodium concentration in the blood, triggering thirst and regulating fluid balance accordingly. It stimulates the release of antidiuretic hormone (ADH or vasopressin) from the posterior pituitary gland to conserve water and maintain electrolyte balance in response to dehydration or changes in blood volume.

6. Circadian Rhythms: The hypothalamus contains the suprachiasmatic nucleus, which serves as the body's internal clock, regulating circadian rhythms such as the sleep-wake cycle, hormone secretion, and body temperature. It receives input from light-sensitive cells in the retina and synchronizes physiological processes with the external environment to ensure optimal timing and coordination.

7. Emotional and Behavioral Responses: Certain regions of the hypothalamus are involved in processing emotional and behavioral responses to stimuli, including fear, aggression, pleasure, and reward. These nuclei integrate sensory inputs and modulate neuroendocrine, autonomic, and behavioral responses to facilitate adaptive reactions to environmental challenges.

8. Reproductive Function: The hypothalamus plays a crucial role in regulating reproductive function by secreting gonadotropin-releasing hormone (GnRH), which stimulates the secretion of gonadotropins (e.g., luteinizing hormone and follicle-stimulating hormone) from the anterior pituitary gland. These hormones control the menstrual cycle, ovulation, spermatogenesis, and sex hormone production, thereby influencing fertility and reproductive health.

3.2 Hypothalamic Hormones and their Regulation

The hypothalamus, a small but crucial region in the brain, serves as the master regulator of the endocrine system by producing a variety of releasing and inhibiting hormones that control the secretion of pituitary hormones. These hypothalamic hormones exert their effects on the anterior pituitary gland through the hypophyseal portal system, a specialized network of blood vessels that connects the hypothalamus and the pituitary gland. Here, we delve into the fine details of the key hypothalamic hormones and their intricate regulatory mechanisms:

Thyrotropin-Releasing Hormone (TRH):

TRH is a tripeptide hormone synthesized and secreted by parvocellular neurons in the paraventricular nucleus of the hypothalamus. It acts on thyrotrophs in the anterior pituitary gland to stimulate the synthesis and release of thyroid-stimulating hormone (TSH). The secretion of TRH is under tight regulation, primarily influenced by negative feedback from thyroid hormones (T3 and T4). When thyroid hormone levels decrease, TRH secretion increases, leading to enhanced TSH release and subsequent stimulation of thyroid hormone synthesis and secretion. Conversely, elevated levels of thyroid hormones inhibit TRH secretion through direct and indirect mechanisms, thereby modulating thyroid function and maintaining hormonal balance.

Gonadotropin-Releasing Hormone (GnRH):

GnRH is a decapeptide hormone synthesized and secreted by neurons in the arcuate nucleus and preoptic area of the hypothalamus. It plays a pivotal role in regulating the secretion of gonadotropins, luteinizing hormone (LH), and follicle-stimulating hormone (FSH), from the anterior pituitary gland. The secretion of GnRH exhibits a characteristic pulsatile pattern, with fluctuations in pulse frequency and amplitude throughout the menstrual cycle and reproductive lifespan. This pulsatile secretion is essential for the regulation of reproductive function, including the timing of ovulation and the menstrual cycle. GnRH secretion is subject to complex regulation by multiple factors, including sex steroids (estrogen and testosterone), neurotransmitters, neuropeptides, and environmental cues. Feedback regulation of GnRH secretion involves both negative and positive feedback mechanisms, with sex steroids exerting inhibitory or stimulatory effects on GnRH release depending on their concentration and temporal patterns.

Corticotropin-Releasing Hormone (CRH):

CRH is a 41-amino acid peptide hormone synthesized and secreted by neurons in the paraventricular nucleus of the hypothalamus. It plays a central role in regulating the body's response to stress by stimulating the secretion of adrenocorticotropic hormone (ACTH) from the anterior pituitary gland. ACTH, in turn, stimulates the synthesis and release of glucocorticoids (e.g., cortisol) from the adrenal cortex. CRH secretion is tightly regulated by a variety of stimuli, including physical, psychological, and environmental stressors. Stress-induced activation of the hypothalamic-pituitary-adrenal (HPA) axis leads to increased CRH release, resulting in enhanced glucocorticoid production and mobilization of energy reserves to cope with the stressor. Negative feedback from glucocorticoids acts to suppress CRH secretion, providing a mechanism for regulating the stress response and preventing excessive glucocorticoid production.

Growth Hormone-Releasing Hormone (GHRH):

GHRH is a 44-amino acid peptide hormone synthesized and secreted by neurons in the arcuate nucleus of the hypothalamus. It stimulates the synthesis and release of growth hormone (GH) from somatotrophs in the anterior pituitary gland. GHRH secretion is regulated by multiple factors, including nutritional status, sleep-wake cycle, exercise, and stress. Ghrelin, a peptide hormone produced by the stomach, acts synergistically with GHRH to stimulate GH release. Negative feedback regulation of GHRH secretion involves GH and insulin-like growth factors (IGFs), with low levels of GH and IGFs stimulating GHRH release and high levels inhibiting GHRH secretion. GHRH pulsatility and amplitude are critical for maintaining normal GH secretion patterns and growth processes throughout life.

Somatostatin (SS):

Somatostatin, also known as growth hormone-inhibiting hormone (GHIH), is a 14-amino acid peptide hormone synthesized and secreted by neurons in the periventricular nucleus and arcuate nucleus of the hypothalamus. It exerts inhibitory effects on the secretion of growth hormone (GH) from somatotrophs in the anterior pituitary gland. Somatostatin also inhibits the secretion of other pituitary hormones, including thyroid-stimulating hormone (TSH), luteinizing hormone (LH), follicle-stimulating hormone (FSH), and adrenocorticotropic hormone (ACTH). Somatostatin secretion is regulated by multiple factors, including GH and IGFs, glucose levels, and neurotransmitters. Negative feedback from GH and IGFs inhibits somatostatin release, whereas low glucose levels and stress can stimulate its secretion. Somatostatin acts locally within the hypothalamus and pituitary gland to modulate hormone secretion patterns and maintain hormonal balance.

3.3 Anatomy and Connectivity of the Hypothalamo-Pituitary Axis:

The hypothalamo-pituitary axis (HPA) is a complex neuroendocrine system that involves the hypothalamus and the pituitary gland, each with distinct anatomical structures and connectivity.

Hypothalamus:

The hypothalamus is a small region located at the base of the brain, below the thalamus and above the pituitary gland. It consists of several nuclei, each with specific functions related to regulating various physiological processes. The paraventricular nucleus (PVN) and the supraoptic nucleus (SON) are particularly important for synthesizing and secreting neurohormones that regulate pituitary function.

Pituitary Gland:

The pituitary gland, also known as the hypophysis, is divided into two distinct lobes: the anterior pituitary (adenohypophysis) and the posterior pituitary (neurohypophysis). It is located at the base of the brain, just below the hypothalamus, and is connected to the hypothalamus via the infundibulum, also known as the pituitary stalk.

- Anterior Pituitary (Adenohypophysis): The anterior pituitary is composed of glandular tissue and synthesizes and secretes several hormones in response to hypothalamic releasing or inhibiting hormones. It receives regulatory signals from the hypothalamus through a specialized system of blood vessels called the hypophyseal portal system.

- Posterior Pituitary (Neurohypophysis): The posterior pituitary is an extension of the hypothalamus and consists of neural tissue. It stores and releases two hormones synthesized in the hypothalamus: oxytocin and vasopressin (antidiuretic hormone). These hormones are transported down axons from the hypothalamus and stored in nerve terminals in the posterior pituitary until they are released into the bloodstream in response to neural signals.

Connectivity:

The hypothalamo-pituitary axis is characterized by intricate connections between the hypothalamus and the pituitary gland, which allow for precise regulation of hormone secretion. These connections include:

- Hypophyseal Portal System: This system consists of a network of blood vessels that connect the hypothalamus to the anterior pituitary gland. Hypothalamic releasing and inhibiting hormones are secreted into capillaries in the median eminence of the hypothalamus, where they are transported via portal veins to the anterior pituitary. Upon reaching the anterior pituitary, these hormones stimulate or inhibit the release of specific pituitary hormones, thereby regulating endocrine function.

- Neural Pathways: Neural connections between the hypothalamus and the posterior pituitary allow for the transport and release of oxytocin and vasopressin synthesized in the hypothalamus. Axons originating from the

PVN and SON project down the infundibulum and terminate in the posterior pituitary, where these hormones are released into the bloodstream in response to neural signals.

Overall, the anatomy and connectivity of the hypothalamo-pituitary axis facilitate the precise regulation of hormone secretion and coordination of physiological processes throughout the body. Dysfunction within this axis can lead to a variety of endocrine disorders, underscoring the importance of understanding its anatomy and function in health and disease.

The function of the hypothalamo-pituitary axis (HPA) is to regulate the secretion of hormones that control various physiological processes within the body. These processes include:

1. Stress Response: One of the primary functions of the HPA axis is to coordinate the body's response to stress. In response to stressors, the hypothalamus releases corticotropin-releasing hormone (CRH), which stimulates the anterior pituitary to produce adrenocorticotropic hormone (ACTH). ACTH, in turn, stimulates the adrenal glands to release cortisol, a stress hormone that mobilizes energy reserves and suppresses inflammation and immune responses.

2. Metabolism: The HPA axis regulates metabolism by influencing the secretion of hormones such as growth hormone (GH), thyroid-stimulating hormone (TSH), and cortisol. GH promotes growth and protein synthesis, while TSH stimulates the thyroid gland to produce thyroid hormones that regulate metabolic rate. Cortisol affects glucose metabolism, lipid metabolism, and protein breakdown, helping to maintain energy balance.

3. Reproduction: The HPA axis plays a crucial role in regulating reproductive function by controlling the secretion of gonadotropin-releasing hormone (GnRH) from the hypothalamus. GnRH stimulates the anterior pituitary to release luteinizing hormone (LH) and follicle-stimulating hormone (FSH), which regulate the menstrual cycle in females and sperm production in males

4. Water Balance: The HPA axis influences water balance and blood pressure through the secretion of vasopressin, also known as antidiuretic hormone (ADH). ADH is produced by the hypothalamus and released by the posterior pituitary in response to changes in blood osmolarity or blood volume. It acts on the kidneys to regulate water reabsorption and maintain blood pressure.

5. Growth and Development: Growth hormone (GH), regulated by the HPA axis, plays a key role in growth and development during childhood and adolescence. GH stimulates the growth of bones and tissues, promotes protein synthesis, and regulates metabolism. Disorders of GH secretion can lead to growth disorders such as dwarfism or gigantism.

Regulation of Hormone Secretion:

The regulation of hormone secretion within the hypothalamo-pituitary axis involves complex interactions between the hypothalamus, the anterior pituitary gland, peripheral endocrine glands, and feedback mechanisms. This process ensures precise control over hormone levels, allowing for the maintenance of physiological homeostasis. Here's a detailed discussion on the regulation of hormone secretion within the hypothalamo-pituitary axis:

1. Hypothalamic-Releasing and Inhibiting Hormones: The hypothalamus synthesizes and releases a variety of hormones that either stimulate or inhibit the secretion of pituitary hormones. These hypothalamic-releasing and inhibiting hormones are transported to the anterior pituitary gland through the hypophyseal portal system, where they exert their effects on specific pituitary cells.

2. Stimulatory Pathways: Corticotropin-Releasing Hormone (CRH): CRH stimulates the secretion of adrenocorticotropic hormone (ACTH) from corticotroph cells in the anterior pituitary. ACTH, in turn, acts on the adrenal cortex to stimulate the synthesis and release of glucocorticoids, such as cortisol. Gonadotropin-Releasing Hormone (GnRH): GnRH regulates the secretion of gonadotropins, including luteinizing hormone (LH) and follicle-stimulating hormone (FSH), from gonadotroph cells in the anterior pituitary. LH and FSH control the function of the gonads and the production of sex hormones (testosterone in males and estrogen in females).

3. Inhibitory Pathways: Somatostatin (SST): Somatostatin, also known as growth hormone-inhibiting hormone (GHIH), inhibits the secretion of growth hormone (GH) from somatotroph cells in the anterior pituitary. Dopamine (DA): Dopamine inhibits the secretion of prolactin from lactotroph cells in the anterior pituitary.

4. Feedback Mechanisms: Negative Feedback: Peripheral hormones, such as cortisol, sex steroids, and thyroid hormones, exert negative feedback on the hypothalamus and anterior pituitary, inhibiting the secretion of hypothalamic-releasing hormones and pituitary tropic hormones. This negative feedback loop helps maintain hormone levels within a narrow physiological range.

Positive Feedback: In certain cases, positive feedback loops can amplify hormone secretion. For example, during childbirth, oxytocin released from the hypothalamus and posterior pituitary stimulates uterine contractions, leading to further oxytocin release until delivery occurs.

5. Diurnal Rhythms and Environmental Cues: Hormone secretion within the hypothalamo-pituitary axis often follows diurnal rhythms, with peaks and troughs occurring at specific times of the day. These rhythms are influenced by internal biological clocks and external factors such as light-dark cycles. Environmental cues, including stress, temperature changes, and nutritional status, can also modulate hormone secretion within the axis. For instance, stressors activate the hypothalamic-pituitary-adrenal (HPA) axis, leading to increased cortisol secretion to cope with the stressor.

3.4 Role of the Hypothalamus in Stress Response

The stress response is a complex physiological reaction that helps the body adapt to challenging situations, known as stressors. The hypothalamus plays a pivotal role in orchestrating this response through activation of the hypothalamic-pituitary-adrenal (HPA) axis, a key neuroendocrine pathway involved in stress regulation.

Activation of the HPA Axis:

When an individual encounters a stressor, whether it's physical, psychological, or environmental, the hypothalamus initiates the stress response by releasing corticotropin-releasing hormone (CRH) into the hypophyseal portal system. CRH travels to the anterior pituitary gland, where it stimulates the secretion of adrenocorticotropic hormone (ACTH) into the bloodstream.

Stimulation of the Adrenal Cortex:

ACTH acts on the adrenal cortex, the outer layer of the adrenal glands located above the kidneys, to induce the synthesis and release of glucocorticoid hormones, primarily cortisol. Cortisol is the body's primary stress hormone and serves numerous functions to help the body cope with stress. It mobilizes energy reserves by increasing glucose production and inhibiting glucose uptake in peripheral tissues, thereby providing the necessary fuel for the body's response to the stressor. Additionally, cortisol suppresses non-essential bodily functions such as immune responses and reproductive processes temporarily, redirecting resources to prioritize survival.

Negative Feedback Regulation:

Once the stressor subsides, cortisol levels decrease, signaling the hypothalamus and pituitary gland to downregulate CRH and ACTH secretion, respectively, through negative feedback mechanisms. This feedback loop helps restore homeostasis and prevent excessive activation of the stress response, which could lead to detrimental effects on health if prolonged or dysregulated.

Impact of Chronic Stress:

Chronic stress, characterized by prolonged exposure to stressful stimuli or situations, can have profound effects on the hypothalamic-pituitary-adrenal (HPA) axis, leading to dysregulation of hormonal responses and disruption of physiological homeostasis. The HPA axis, which normally serves to coordinate the body's response to stress, becomes overactivated or dysregulated in the face of chronic stressors, contributing to the development and progression of various physical and mental health disorders.

Persistent Activation of the HPA Axis: Chronic stress triggers sustained activation of the HPA axis, resulting in elevated levels of glucocorticoids, such as cortisol, in the bloodstream. This prolonged exposure to glucocorticoids can have deleterious effects on multiple organ systems, including the cardiovascular, immune, and central nervous systems.

Impaired Negative Feedback Mechanisms: Under normal conditions, circulating glucocorticoids exert negative feedback on the hypothalamus and pituitary gland, inhibiting further release of corticotropin-releasing hormone (CRH) and adrenocorticotropic hormone (ACTH), respectively. However, chronic stress can disrupt these feedback mechanisms, leading to impaired sensitivity of glucocorticoid receptors and reduced effectiveness of negative feedback inhibition. As a result, cortisol levels may remain elevated despite the presence of high glucocorticoid concentrations, perpetuating the cycle of HPA axis activation.

Altered Neurotransmitter and Neuropeptide Levels: Chronic stress can also lead to dysregulation of neurotransmitter and neuropeptide systems within the brain, including alterations in serotonin, dopamine, and neuropeptide Y levels. These changes can affect mood, behavior, and stress responsiveness, contributing to the development of mood disorders such as depression and anxiety.

Immune System Dysregulation: Prolonged exposure to elevated glucocorticoid levels can suppress immune function and increase susceptibility to infections, inflammatory conditions, and autoimmune diseases. Chronic stress-induced immunosuppression can impair the body's ability to mount an effective immune response, leading to increased risk of illness and delayed recovery from infections.

Metabolic and Cardiovascular Effects: Dysregulation of the HPA axis and prolonged elevation of glucocorticoids can also have adverse effects on metabolism and cardiovascular function. Chronic stress-induced hypercortisolemia is associated with insulin resistance, abdominal obesity, dyslipidemia, hypertension, and increased risk of cardiovascular disease.

Psychological and Behavioral Consequences: Chronic stress is strongly associated with the development of psychological disorders, including depression, anxiety, post-traumatic stress disorder (PTSD), and substance abuse disorders. Behavioral changes such as altered sleep patterns, appetite disturbances, social withdrawal, and impaired cognitive function may also occur in response to chronic stressors.

3.5 Conclusion

This chapter examined the crucial role of the endocrine hypothalamus in regulating the body's hormonal balance. We explored its anatomy and location, highlighting its function as a bridge between the nervous and endocrine systems. Key hypothalamic hormones, such as TRH and CRH, were discussed, along with their roles in controlling the anterior and posterior pituitary glands.

We focused on the hypothalamic-pituitary axis and the feedback mechanisms that ensure precise hormone regulation. Understanding these processes is vital for grasping how the body maintains homeostasis and for diagnosing and treating hypothalamic disorders.

This chapter provides a foundational understanding of the hypothalamus's role, preparing us for deeper exploration of specific endocrine glands and their functions in the following chapters.

Case Studies

Case Study 1: Hypothalamic Dysfunction and Pituitary Regulation

Patient Profile:

- Name: Sarah Johnson

- Age: 32 years

- Sex: Female

- Occupation: Teacher

- Medical History: History of headaches, occasional vision disturbances

- Family History: No significant endocrine disorders

Presentation:

Sarah presents to the clinic with complaints of persistent headaches, irregular menstrual cycles, and recent weight gain. She reports feeling fatigued despite adequate sleep and has noted some vision problems, particularly peripheral vision loss.

Physical Examination:

- Vital Signs: BP: 120/80 mmHg, HR: 70 bpm, Temp: 37°C

- Neurological Examination: Normal reflexes, some difficulty with peripheral vision

- Endocrine Examination: Normal thyroid palpation, no palpable masses

Laboratory Tests:

- Serum Cortisol: Low

- ACTH (Adrenocorticotropic Hormone): Low

- TSH (Thyroid-Stimulating Hormone): Low-normal

- Prolactin: Elevated

- MRI of Brain: Enlarged pituitary gland with possible compression of optic chiasm

Discussion:

Sarah's symptoms, lab results, and MRI findings suggest a hypothalamic or pituitary disorder, potentially a pituitary adenoma causing compression of the optic chiasm and affecting the secretion of multiple pituitary hormones.

Questions:

1. Explain the role of the hypothalamus in regulating pituitary function.

2. What are the potential causes of Sarah's symptoms related to hypothalamic dysfunction?

3. How does hypothalamic-pituitary axis dysfunction affect hormonal balance?

4. Discuss the clinical significance of elevated prolactin levels in Sarah's case.

Case Study 2: Hypothalamic-Pituitary-Adrenal Axis Dysfunction

Patient Profile:

- Name: Michael Brown

- Age: 40 years

- Sex: Male

- Occupation: Engineer

- Medical History: Depression, chronic fatigue

- Family History: Father had Addison's disease

Presentation:

Michael reports persistent fatigue, low mood, and weight loss over the past six months. He mentions difficulty waking up in the morning and a decreased appetite. His primary care physician referred him to an endocrinologist after initial blood tests showed abnormalities.

Physical Examination:

- Vital Signs: BP: 110/70 mmHg, HR: 65 bpm, Temp: 36.5°C

- General Appearance: Thin, pale, appears tired

- Endocrine Examination: Normal

Laboratory Tests:

- Serum Cortisol: Very low

- ACTH (Adrenocorticotropic Hormone): Elevated

- Electrolytes: Low sodium, high potassium

- 24-hour Urine Free Cortisol: Low

Discussion:

Michael's symptoms and laboratory results indicate primary adrenal insufficiency (Addison's disease). The elevated ACTH and low cortisol levels suggest that the hypothalamus and pituitary are functioning correctly, but the adrenal glands are not responding appropriately.

Questions:

1. Describe the role of the hypothalamus in the regulation of the adrenal glands.

2. What mechanisms could lead to elevated ACTH levels in Michael's case?

3. How does the feedback loop involving cortisol and ACTH operate under normal conditions?

4. Explain the significance of Michael's electrolyte imbalances in the context of his endocrine disorder.

Practice Questions for Self-Assessment

Multiple Choice Questions

1. Which hormone is directly released by the hypothalamus to stimulate the anterior pituitary?

   a) Thyroid-stimulating hormone (TSH)

   b) Corticotropin-releasing hormone (CRH)

   c) Adrenocorticotropic hormone (ACTH)

   d) Prolactin

2. The hypothalamus primarily communicates with the anterior pituitary through:

   a) Neural connections

   b) Blood vessels in the hypophyseal portal system

   c) Direct hormone release into the bloodstream

   d) Cerebrospinal fluid

3. Which of the following hormones is NOT released by the anterior pituitary?

   a) Growth hormone (GH)

   b) Prolactin

   c) Oxytocin

   d) Follicle-stimulating hormone (FSH)

4. A tumor in the hypothalamus that inhibits TRH production would likely cause:

   a) Elevated TSH and thyroid hormone levels

   b) Low TSH and elevated thyroid hormone levels

   c) Low TSH and low thyroid hormone levels

   d) Elevated TSH and low thyroid hormone levels

5. Which hormone regulates water balance and is released by the posterior pituitary?

a) Antidiuretic hormone (ADH)

b) Luteinizing hormone (LH)

c) Adrenocorticotropic hormone (ACTH)

d) Growth hormone (GH)

Short Answer Questions

1. Describe the role of the hypothalamus in endocrine regulation.

2. Explain how the hypothalamus communicates with the anterior and posterior pituitary glands.

3. Discuss the importance of the hypothalamic-pituitary axis in maintaining homeostasis.

4. Describe the impact of hypothalamic lesions on pituitary hormone secretion.

5. Explain how hypothalamic dysfunction can lead to multiple endocrine disorders.

True or False Questions

1. The hypothalamus directly secretes thyroid-stimulating hormone (TSH). (True/False)

2. The hypothalamus and posterior pituitary gland are connected by neural pathways. (True/False)

3. Corticotropin-releasing hormone (CRH) stimulates the release of ACTH from the anterior pituitary. (True/False)

4. Hypothalamic dysfunction can lead to secondary adrenal insufficiency. (True/False)

5. The hypothalamus is involved in regulating circadian rhythms. (True/False)

Answers

Case Study 1

1. Role of the Hypothalamus in Pituitary Function:

- The hypothalamus regulates pituitary function by releasing hormones that either stimulate or inhibit the release of pituitary hormones. It produces releasing hormones like TRH, CRH, GnRH, and GHRH that stimulate the anterior pituitary and inhibitory hormones like somatostatin and dopamine.

2. Causes of Sarah's Symptoms:

- Sarah's symptoms could be due to a pituitary adenoma causing compression and disrupting hormone production, leading to deficiencies in ACTH, TSH, and other pituitary hormones. The compression of the optic chiasm explains her vision disturbances.

3. Hypothalamic-Pituitary Axis Dysfunction:

- Dysfunction in the hypothalamic-pituitary axis can disrupt the secretion of multiple hormones, leading to a cascade of hormonal imbalances. For instance, insufficient CRH leads to low ACTH and cortisol, causing symptoms like fatigue and weight gain.

4. Elevated Prolactin Levels:

- Elevated prolactin in Sarah's case could indicate a prolactinoma, a pituitary tumor that secretes prolactin. High prolactin levels can cause menstrual irregularities, galactorrhea, and infertility. It may also inhibit the release of GnRH, affecting other hormonal pathways.

Case Study 2

1. Role of Hypothalamus in Adrenal Regulation:

- The hypothalamus regulates adrenal function through the release of CRH, which stimulates the anterior pituitary to secrete ACTH. ACTH then stimulates the adrenal cortex to produce cortisol, which is vital for stress response and metabolic functions.

2. Mechanisms Leading to Elevated ACTH:

- Elevated ACTH levels in Michael's case indicate primary adrenal insufficiency (Addison's disease). The adrenal glands fail to produce cortisol, prompting the hypothalamus and pituitary to increase CRH and ACTH production in an attempt to stimulate cortisol synthesis.

3. Cortisol-ACTH Feedback Loop:

- Under normal conditions, cortisol exerts negative feedback on the hypothalamus and pituitary, inhibiting CRH and ACTH production. This feedback loop maintains cortisol levels within a narrow range, ensuring appropriate responses to stress and metabolic demands.

4. Significance of Electrolyte Imbalances:

- Michael's low sodium and high potassium levels are characteristic of Addison's disease, where aldosterone deficiency leads to impaired sodium retention and potassium excretion. This imbalance can cause symptoms like fatigue, low blood pressure, and dehydration.

Multiple Choice Questions

1. b) Corticotropin-releasing hormone (CRH)

2. b) Blood vessels in the hypophyseal portal system

3. c) Oxytocin

4. c) Low TSH and low thyroid hormone levels

5. a) Antidiuretic hormone (ADH)

Short Answer Questions

1. Role of the Hypothalamus:

- The hypothalamus regulates endocrine function by producing releasing and inhibiting hormones that control the secretion of pituitary hormones. It integrates neural and endocrine signals to maintain homeostasis and coordinate bodily functions.

2. Hypothalamic Communication with Pituitary Glands:

- The hypothalamus communicates with the anterior pituitary via the hypophyseal portal system, a network of blood vessels that carry releasing and inhibiting hormones directly to the anterior pituitary. It communicates with the posterior pituitary via neural connections, where hypothalamic neurons release hormones directly into the bloodstream.

3. Hypothalamic-Pituitary Axis in Homeostasis:

- The hypothalamic-pituitary axis is crucial for maintaining homeostasis by regulating various endocrine glands and their hormone production. It ensures proper growth, metabolism, stress response, and reproductive functions.

4. Impact of Hypothalamic Lesions:

- Lesions in the hypothalamus can disrupt the release of releasing or inhibiting hormones, leading to deficiencies or excesses in pituitary hormones. This can cause disorders such as hypopituitarism, where multiple hormone levels are affected.

5. Hypothalamic Dysfunction and Endocrine Disorders:

- Hypothalamic dysfunction can lead to secondary endocrine disorders due to impaired regulation of pituitary hormones. Examples include secondary adrenal insufficiency, hypothyroidism, and gonadal dysfunction, resulting in symptoms like fatigue, metabolic imbalances, and reproductive issues.

True or False Questions

1. False

2. True

3. True

4. True

5. True

Bibliography

1. Ganong, W. F. (2005). Review of Medical Physiology (22nd ed.). McGraw-Hill Medical.

   - This textbook provides a comprehensive overview of endocrine physiology, including detailed sections on the hypothalamus and its role in hormonal regulation.

2. Guyton, A. C., & Hall, J. E. (2016). Textbook of Medical Physiology (13th ed.). Saunders.

   - This authoritative textbook discusses the physiological principles of the hypothalamus, emphasizing its integration in the regulation of endocrine functions.

3. Moore, K. L., & Agur, A. M. R. (2014). Essential Clinical Anatomy (5th ed.). Lippincott Williams & Wilkins.

   - Offers anatomical insights into the hypothalamus, essential for understanding its structural basis and connection with the pituitary gland.

4. Krieger, D. T. (1994). Brain Peptides and Pituitary Function. Springer Science & Business Media.

   - Focuses on the neuroendocrine aspects of the hypothalamus, detailing its peptide hormones and their role in regulating pituitary hormone secretion.

5. Kalra, S. P. (Ed.). (2017). Hypothalamus in Health and Diseases. Elsevier.

   - Provides in-depth reviews on the hypothalamus, covering its anatomy, physiology, and clinical relevance in various health conditions.

Chapter 4

Physiology of Adenohypophyseal (Anterior Pituitary) System

4.1 Anatomy and Structure of Adenohypophysis:

The adenohypophysis, or anterior pituitary gland, is a small, pea-sized structure located at the base of the brain, beneath the hypothalamus, and above the posterior pituitary gland. It is connected to the hypothalamus by a complex network of blood vessels known as the hypophyseal portal system. This portal system allows for the direct communication between the hypothalamus and the anterior pituitary, facilitating the regulation of hormone secretion.

Anatomy:

The adenohypophysis can be anatomically divided into three distinct regions:

1. Pars Distalis:

- The pars distalis, or anterior lobe, is the largest and most functionally significant region of the adenohypophysis.

- It consists of various cell types organized into clusters or cords separated by fenestrated capillaries.

- These cells include somatotrophs, lactotrophs, thyrotrophs, corticotrophs, and gonadotrophs, each of which produces specific hormones.

2. Pars Intermedia:

- The pars intermedia is a narrow zone of cells located between the pars distalis and the posterior pituitary.

- In humans, it is relatively inconspicuous and less functionally significant compared to other species.

- It produces melanocyte-stimulating hormone (MSH) in some vertebrates but is rudimentary and functionally inactive in humans.

3. Pars Tuberalis:

- The pars tuberalis is a thin layer of cells that wraps around the infundibulum, the stalk-like structure connecting the pituitary gland to the hypothalamus.

- It plays a role in regulating the secretion of certain hormones, particularly those involved in seasonal reproductive cycles.

Cell Types:

Within the pars distalis, several distinct cell types can be identified based on their morphology and hormone production:

1. Somatotrophs:

   - Somatotrophs are the most abundant cell type in the adenohypophysis.

   - They produce and secrete growth hormone (GH), also known as somatotropin, which regulates growth and metabolism.

2. Lactotrophs:

   - Lactotrophs are responsible for the synthesis and secretion of prolactin (PRL).

   - Prolactin stimulates milk production (lactation) in the mammary glands of females and has various roles in reproductive function and behavior.

3. Thyrotrophs:

   - Thyrotrophs produce thyroid-stimulating hormone (TSH), also known as thyrotropin.

   - TSH stimulates the thyroid gland to produce and release thyroid hormones (thyroxine T4 and triiodothyronine T3), which regulate metabolism and energy expenditure.

4. Corticotrophs:

   - Corticotrophs secrete adrenocorticotropic hormone (ACTH), also known as corticotropin.

   - ACTH stimulates the adrenal cortex to produce and release glucocorticoids, primarily cortisol, which play a key role in the body's response to stress and inflammation.

5. Gonadotrophs:

   - Gonadotrophs produce two gonadotropic hormones: luteinizing hormone (LH) and follicle-stimulating hormone (FSH).

   - LH and FSH regulate gonadal function and reproductive processes in both males and females, including gametogenesis (spermatogenesis and oogenesis) and sex hormone secretion (testosterone, estrogen, and progesterone).

4.2 Hormones Produced by Adenohypophysis:

The adenohypophysis, or anterior pituitary gland, is a crucial endocrine organ responsible for synthesizing and secreting several hormones that regulate various physiological processes throughout the body. Here, we will explore each hormone produced by the adenohypophysis, its structure, synthesis, regulation, and physiological functions:

Growth Hormone (GH):

Structure: Growth hormone is a peptide hormone composed of 191 amino acids.

Synthesis: GH is synthesized and secreted by somatotroph cells located primarily in the pars distalis of the adenohypophysis.

Regulation: GH secretion is regulated by the hypothalamic peptide hormone, growth hormone-releasing hormone (GHRH), which stimulates GH synthesis and secretion. Conversely, somatostatin (growth hormone-inhibiting hormone), released by the hypothalamus, inhibits GH secretion.

Physiological Functions: GH promotes growth and development by stimulating cell proliferation, differentiation, and elongation, particularly in bone and muscle tissues. It enhances protein synthesis, lipolysis, and the mobilization of fatty acids, contributing to increased lean body mass and energy expenditure. GH also plays a role in glucose metabolism by promoting gluconeogenesis and reducing glucose uptake in peripheral tissues, thus maintaining blood glucose levels.

Prolactin (PRL):

Structure: Prolactin is a peptide hormone consisting of a single polypeptide chain.

Synthesis: PRL is produced by lactotroph cells in the adenohypophysis.

Regulation: PRL secretion is primarily under inhibitory control by dopamine (prolactin-inhibitory hormone), released by the hypothalamus. Prolactin-releasing hormone (PRH), also synthesized by the hypothalamus, stimulates PRL secretion but is of lesser physiological significance.

Physiological Functions: PRL promotes mammary gland development and lactation in females by stimulating milk production and secretion. It also influences reproductive function by suppressing gonadotropin-releasing hormone (GnRH) secretion, leading to inhibition of ovulation and menstruation during lactation.

Thyroid-Stimulating Hormone (TSH):

Structure: Thyroid-stimulating hormone is a glycoprotein hormone composed of alpha and beta subunits.

Synthesis: TSH is synthesized by thyrotroph cells in the adenohypophysis.

Regulation: TSH secretion is regulated by thyrotropin-releasing hormone (TRH), released by the hypothalamus in response to low thyroid hormone levels. Negative feedback from circulating thyroid hormones (T3 and T4) inhibits TRH and TSH secretion when thyroid hormone levels are elevated.

Physiological Functions: TSH stimulates the synthesis and secretion of thyroid hormones (T3 and T4) by the thyroid gland, which are essential for regulating metabolic rate, energy expenditure, and tissue growth and development.

Adrenocorticotropic Hormone (ACTH):

Structure: Adrenocorticotropic hormone is a peptide hormone composed of 39 amino acids.

Synthesis: ACTH is produced by corticotroph cells in the adenohypophysis.

Regulation: ACTH secretion is primarily regulated by corticotropin-releasing hormone (CRH), released by the hypothalamus in response to stress, low blood glucose levels, and diurnal rhythm. Negative feedback from glucocorticoids (e.g., cortisol) inhibits CRH and ACTH secretion when cortisol levels are elevated.

Physiological Functions: ACTH stimulates the synthesis and secretion of glucocorticoids, primarily cortisol, by the adrenal cortex in response to stress, inflammation, and other physiological stimuli.

Luteinizing Hormone (LH) and Follicle-Stimulating Hormone (FSH):

Structure: LH and FSH are glycoprotein hormones composed of alpha and beta subunits.

Synthesis: LH and FSH are produced by gonadotroph cells in the adenohypophysis.

Regulation: Gonadotropin-releasing hormone (GnRH), released by the hypothalamus, regulates the secretion of LH and FSH in a pulsatile manner. Feedback from gonadal steroids (e.g., estrogen, progesterone, testosterone) modulates GnRH, LH, and FSH secretion through negative feedback loops.

Physiological Functions: LH stimulates ovulation, corpus luteum formation, and synthesis of sex hormones (e.g., estrogen, progesterone in females; testosterone in males). FSH promotes follicular development in the ovaries and spermatogenesis in the testes, contributing to reproductive function in both sexes.

4.3 Regulation of Adenohypophyseal Hormones:

The secretion of hormones by the adenohypophysis is intricately regulated by a combination of hypothalamic, peripheral, and feedback mechanisms, ensuring precise control over endocrine function and maintaining homeostasis within the body. This regulation involves the interplay between hypothalamic releasing and inhibitory hormones, peripheral hormones, and feedback loops.

Hypothalamic Control:

The hypothalamus, a crucial neuroendocrine organ located above the pituitary gland, exerts primary control over adenohypophyseal hormone secretion through the release of specific regulatory factors. These factors are secreted into the hypophyseal portal system, a network of blood vessels that directly connects the hypothalamus and adenohypophysis.

1. Hypothalamic Releasing Hormones:

Various hypothalamic releasing hormones stimulate the synthesis and secretion of specific adenohypophyseal hormones. For example, growth hormone-releasing hormone (GHRH) stimulates the release of growth hormone (GH), thyrotropin-releasing hormone (TRH) stimulates thyroid-stimulating hormone (TSH) secretion, and gonadotropin-releasing hormone (GnRH) regulates the secretion of luteinizing hormone (LH) and follicle-stimulating hormone (FSH).

2. Hypothalamic Inhibitory Hormones:

Conversely, the hypothalamus also produces inhibitory hormones that suppress adenohypophyseal hormone secretion. Somatostatin, also known as growth hormone-inhibiting hormone (GHIH), inhibits the release of GH, while dopamine inhibits the secretion of prolactin (PRL).

Peripheral Regulation:

In addition to hypothalamic control, peripheral hormones and physiological factors influence adenohypophyseal hormone secretion.

Peripheral hormones, such as thyroid hormones (T3 and T4), adrenal steroids (cortisol), and gonadal hormones (estrogen, testosterone), exert feedback effects on the hypothalamus and adenohypophysis. For example, elevated levels of thyroid hormones inhibit the secretion of TRH and TSH through a negative feedback loop, regulating thyroid function.

Feedback Mechanisms:

Feedback loops play a critical role in fine-tuning hormone secretion and maintaining hormonal balance within the body.

1. Negative Feedback:

Negative feedback loops involve the inhibition of hormone secretion in response to elevated hormone levels, maintaining physiological equilibrium. For instance, high levels of cortisol inhibit the release of corticotropin-releasing hormone (CRH) from the hypothalamus and ACTH from the adenohypophysis, regulating the body's stress response.

2. Positive Feedback:

Positive feedback loops amplify hormonal responses, leading to increased hormone secretion. An example of positive feedback is the surge in LH secretion triggered by rising estrogen levels during the menstrual cycle, ultimately culminating in ovulation.

4.4 Conclusion

In conclusion, this chapter has provided a comprehensive overview of the physiology of the adenohypophyseal (anterior pituitary) system, highlighting its critical role in regulating numerous physiological processes through the secretion of various hormones. The adenohypophysis, located at the base of the brain, consists of distinct cell types that produce hormones such as growth hormone, prolactin, thyroid-stimulating hormone, adrenocorticotropic hormone, and gonadotropins.

The regulation of adenohypophyseal hormone secretion is tightly controlled by hypothalamic releasing and inhibitory hormones, as well as feedback mechanisms from peripheral hormones. This intricate regulatory network ensures hormonal balance and homeostasis within the body.

The functions of adenohypophyseal hormones are diverse and include the regulation of growth and development, reproduction, and metabolism. These hormones play essential roles in maintaining overall health and wellbeing.

By understanding the anatomy, hormone production, regulation, and functions of the adenohypophysis, we gain valuable insights into the complex interplay between the endocrine system and other organ systems. Further exploration of specific adenohypophyseal hormones and their effects on target tissues will enhance our understanding of endocrine physiology and its implications for health and disease.

Case Studies

Case Study 1: Growth Hormone Dysregulation

Patient Profile:

- Name: Robert Jones

- Age: 52 years

- Sex: Male

- Occupation: Construction Worker

- Medical History: Hypertension, history of joint pain

- Family History: No known endocrine disorders

Presentation:

Robert presents with complaints of increased hand and foot size, coarse facial features, and joint pain. He has noticed that his rings and shoes no longer fit. He also reports headaches and visual disturbances.

Physical Examination:

- Vital Signs: BP: 150/95 mmHg, HR: 70 bpm, Temp: 36.7°C

- General Appearance: Enlarged hands and feet, prominent jaw, and thickened skin

- Neurological Examination: Bitemporal hemianopia (loss of peripheral vision)

Laboratory Tests:

- Serum IGF-1 (Insulin-like Growth Factor 1): Elevated

- Growth Hormone (GH) levels: Elevated

- Oral Glucose Tolerance Test (OGTT): Failure of GH suppression

Imaging:

- MRI Brain: Pituitary macroadenoma

Discussion:

Robert's presentation and laboratory findings suggest acromegaly, a condition caused by excessive GH secretion, often due to a pituitary adenoma. The enlarged pituitary gland can compress the optic chiasm, leading to visual disturbances.

Questions:

1. Describe the physiological role of growth hormone (GH) and its regulation.

2. Explain how a pituitary adenoma can lead to the symptoms observed in Robert.

3. Discuss the relationship between GH and IGF-1 in the context of acromegaly.

4. What are the long-term complications of untreated acromegaly?

Case Study 2: Hypopituitarism

Patient Profile:

- Name: Emily Davis

- Age: 30 years

- Sex: Female

- Occupation: Teacher

- Medical History: Severe postpartum hemorrhage one year ago

Presentation:

Emily presents with fatigue, weight loss, loss of appetite, and amenorrhea (absence of menstruation). She reports feeling cold all the time and has noted thinning of her hair. She also mentions that she has not been able to produce breast milk since her childbirth.

Physical Examination:

- Vital Signs: BP: 100/65 mmHg, HR: 55 bpm, Temp: 35.9°C

- General Appearance: Appears tired and pale

- Skin and Hair: Dry skin, thinning hair

Laboratory Tests:

- Cortisol: Low

- TSH (Thyroid-Stimulating Hormone): Low

- Free T4: Low

- LH (Luteinizing Hormone) and FSH (Follicle-Stimulating Hormone): Low

- Prolactin: Low

Imaging:

- MRI Brain: Small pituitary gland

Discussion:

Emily's symptoms and lab results suggest hypopituitarism, likely due to Sheehan's syndrome, which occurs due to pituitary gland necrosis following severe postpartum hemorrhage. The deficiency of multiple pituitary hormones is causing her symptoms.

Questions:

1. Explain the role of the anterior pituitary hormones affected in Emily's case.

2. Discuss how Sheehan's syndrome can lead to hypopituitarism.

3. Describe the clinical manifestations of hypopituitarism.

4. What are the treatment options for Emily's condition?

Practice Questions for Self-Assessment

Multiple Choice Questions

1. Which hormone is primarily responsible for stimulating the release of growth hormone (GH) from the anterior pituitary?

   a) Thyrotropin-releasing hormone (TRH)

   b) Corticotropin-releasing hormone (CRH)

   c) Growth hormone-releasing hormone (GHRH)

   d) Gonadotropin-releasing hormone (GnRH)

2. Which of the following conditions is characterized by an excess of adrenocorticotropic hormone (ACTH)?

   a) Cushing's disease

   b) Addison's disease

   c) Hypothyroidism

   d) Diabetes insipidus

3. Which hormone is produced by the anterior pituitary and stimulates the adrenal cortex?

   a) TSH

   b) ACTH

   c) LH

   d) FSH

4. Which of the following is a symptom of prolactinoma?

   a) Hyperthyroidism

   b) Galactorrhea (milk production)

   c) Cushingoid features

   d) Hyperpigmentation

5. The primary function of follicle-stimulating hormone (FSH) is to:

   a) Stimulate ovulation

   b) Stimulate milk production

c) Stimulate adrenal cortex activity

d) Stimulate gamete production

Short Answer Questions

1. Describe the role of the hypothalamus in regulating anterior pituitary function.

2. Explain the physiological effects of adrenocorticotropic hormone (ACTH).

3. Discuss the feedback mechanisms involved in the regulation of thyroid-stimulating hormone (TSH).

4. What is the role of luteinizing hormone (LH) in the reproductive system?

5. Describe the clinical presentation of a patient with a prolactinoma.

True or False Questions

1. The anterior pituitary produces oxytocin. (True/False)

2. Growth hormone has both direct and indirect effects on tissues. (True/False)

3. Hypersecretion of ACTH can lead to adrenal insufficiency. (True/False)

4. Prolactin is primarily regulated by dopamine from the hypothalamus. (True/False)

5. FSH and LH are collectively referred to as gonadotropins. (True/False)

Answers

Case Study 1

1. Physiological Role of Growth Hormone (GH) and Its Regulation:

- GH promotes growth and development by stimulating protein synthesis and cell growth. It increases bone and muscle mass and influences metabolism by increasing lipolysis and decreasing glucose uptake. GH secretion is regulated by growth hormone-releasing hormone (GHRH) and somatostatin from the hypothalamus, as well as feedback from IGF-1 levels.

2. Pituitary Adenoma and Symptoms in Robert:

- A pituitary adenoma can secrete excessive GH, leading to acromegaly. The tumor's growth can compress nearby structures, such as the optic chiasm, causing visual disturbances like bitemporal hemianopia. Excess GH causes enlarged bones and tissues, resulting in the characteristic features of acromegaly.

3. Relationship Between GH and IGF-1 in Acromegaly:

- GH stimulates the liver and other tissues to produce IGF-1, which mediates many of GH's growth-promoting effects. In acromegaly, elevated GH levels lead to increased IGF-1 production, contributing to tissue overgrowth and metabolic disturbances.

4. Long-term Complications of Untreated Acromegaly:

- Untreated acromegaly can lead to severe joint problems, cardiovascular diseases, diabetes mellitus, sleep apnea, and increased risk of certain cancers. Early diagnosis and treatment are crucial to prevent these complications.

Case Study 2

1. Role of Anterior Pituitary Hormones in Emily's Case:

- The anterior pituitary secretes hormones such as ACTH, TSH, LH, FSH, and prolactin, which regulate adrenal function, thyroid activity, reproductive function, and lactation. Deficiency in these hormones leads to symptoms like fatigue, weight loss, amenorrhea, and inability to lactate.

2. Sheehan's Syndrome and Hypopituitarism:

- Sheehan's syndrome occurs due to ischemic necrosis of the pituitary gland following severe postpartum hemorrhage. This leads to hypopituitarism, characterized by a deficiency in one or more anterior pituitary hormones, affecting multiple endocrine functions.

3. Clinical Manifestations of Hypopituitarism:

- Symptoms include fatigue, weight loss, low blood pressure, cold intolerance, amenorrhea, infertility, decreased libido, and hair loss. These symptoms result from deficiencies in cortisol, thyroid hormones, sex hormones, and other pituitary hormones.

4. Treatment Options for Hypopituitarism:

- Treatment involves hormone replacement therapy to address deficiencies. This may include corticosteroids for adrenal insufficiency, levothyroxine for hypothyroidism, sex hormone replacement (estrogen/progesterone for women, testosterone for men), and possibly growth hormone if needed.

Multiple Choice Questions

1. c) Growth hormone-releasing hormone (GHRH)

2. a) Cushing's disease

3. b) ACTH

4. b) Galactorrhea (milk production)

5. d) Stimulate gamete production

Short Answer Questions

1. Hypothalamus and Anterior Pituitary Function:

- The hypothalamus regulates anterior pituitary function through releasing and inhibiting hormones. It secretes hormones like TRH, CRH, GHRH, GnRH, and somatostatin, which travel to the anterior pituitary via the hypophyseal portal system, stimulating or inhibiting the release of pituitary hormones.

2. Physiological Effects of ACTH:

- ACTH stimulates the adrenal cortex to produce and release cortisol, which helps regulate metabolism, immune response, and stress response. ACTH also promotes the production of adrenal androgens and aldosterone to a lesser extent.

3. Feedback Mechanisms in TSH Regulation:

- TSH release is stimulated by TRH from the hypothalamus. Elevated thyroid hormone levels (T3 and T4) provide negative feedback to the hypothalamus and pituitary, reducing TRH and TSH secretion, maintaining hormonal balance.

4. Role of Luteinizing Hormone (LH) in Reproductive System:

- In females, LH triggers ovulation and stimulates the production of estrogen and progesterone from the ovaries. In males, LH stimulates Leydig cells in the testes to produce testosterone, essential for spermatogenesis and secondary sexual characteristics.

5. Clinical Presentation of Prolactinoma:

- Prolactinomas, benign tumors of the pituitary gland, cause hypersecretion of prolactin. Symptoms include galactorrhea, amenorrhea, infertility, and hypogonadism. In men, symptoms may include decreased libido, erectile dysfunction, and gynecomastia.

True or False Questions

1. False

2. True

3. False

4. True

5. True

Bibliography

1. Alberts, B., Johnson, A., Lewis, J., Raff, M., Roberts, K., & Walter, P. (2002). Molecular Biology of the Cell (4th ed.). Garland Science.

   - This textbook provides in-depth coverage of cellular and molecular biology, including chapters on endocrine signaling pathways and hormone secretion mechanisms.

2. Melmed, S., Polonsky, K. S., Larsen, P. R., & Kronenberg, H. M. (2016). Williams Textbook of Endocrinology (13th ed.). Elsevier.

   - A comprehensive reference covering all aspects of endocrinology, including detailed sections on pituitary anatomy, physiology, and hormone secretion.

3. Fliers, E., & Romijn, J. A. (2007). Regulation of pituitary hormone secretion: Implications for the regulation of body composition. European Journal of Endocrinology, 157(Suppl 1), S21-S29.

   - This review article discusses the complex regulatory mechanisms involved in pituitary hormone secretion, focusing on the interactions between the hypothalamus and anterior pituitary.

4. Shupnik, M. A. (2006). Growth hormone signaling pathways. Growth Hormone & IGF Research, 16(1), 1-11.

   - An article that explores the signaling pathways involved in growth hormone action, relevant to the discussion of adenohypophyseal hormones and their effects.

5. Kaiser, U. B., & Conn, P. M. (2007). The molecular and cellular basis of gonadotropin-releasing hormone action in the pituitary and hypothalamus. Endocrine Reviews, 28(7), 811-877.

   - Although focused on gonadotropin-releasing hormone, this review provides insights into general mechanisms of hypothalamic-pituitary interactions, relevant to understanding adenohypophyseal regulation.

Chapter Five

Physiology of Neurohypophyseal System (Posterior Pituitary)

The neurohypophysis, also known as the posterior pituitary, plays a vital role in the regulation of several physiological processes through the release of two key hormones: oxytocin and vasopressin (antidiuretic hormone, ADH). This chapter will provide a detailed overview of the anatomy, synthesis, secretion, functions, and regulation of the neurohypophyseal hormones.

5.1 Anatomy and Structure of the Neurohypophyseal System:

The neurohypophysis, also known as the posterior pituitary, is a critical component of the pituitary gland, located at the base of the brain below the hypothalamus. Its anatomy and structure are essential for understanding its functions in hormone storage and release, as well as its intricate connections with the hypothalamus and the broader endocrine system.

Location and Connections:

The neurohypophysis is situated at the posterior portion of the pituitary gland, adjacent to the hypothalamus. Its close proximity to the hypothalamus facilitates the communication and integration of signals between these two structures. The neurohypophysis is connected to the hypothalamus via the pituitary stalk or infundibulum, a conduit through which hypothalamic neurons extend their axons to reach the posterior pituitary. This anatomical arrangement allows for the direct transmission of neuroendocrine signals from the hypothalamus to the posterior pituitary, where hormones are stored and released into the bloodstream.

Histological Composition:

Unlike the anterior pituitary, which contains glandular cells known as adenohypophysis, the neurohypophysis primarily consists of nerve fibers, axon terminals, and glial cells. The nerve fibers originate from neurons located in the hypothalamus, specifically the supraoptic and paraventricular nuclei. These neurons project their axons through the pituitary stalk and terminate in the posterior pituitary, forming neurosecretory endings. Glial cells, particularly pituicytes, are supportive cells found within the neurohypophysis. Pituicytes provide structural support and help maintain the extracellular environment necessary for neuronal function.

Nerve Fibers and Terminals:

The supraoptic and paraventricular nuclei of the hypothalamus give rise to distinct populations of neurons that project their axons to the neurohypophysis. These axons contain secretory vesicles filled with neurohypophyseal hormones, namely oxytocin and vasopressin. The axons travel through the pituitary stalk and terminate in the posterior pituitary, where they release their secretory products into the bloodstream in response to specific stimuli. The release of hormones from the neurohypophysis is regulated by neuronal impulses originating in the hypothalamus, which integrate various sensory and physiological inputs.

Vascular Supply:

The neurohypophysis receives its blood supply from the superior hypophyseal artery, a branch of the internal carotid artery. Capillary networks within the neurohypophysis allow for the exchange of hormones between the bloodstream and axon terminals of hypothalamic neurons. This vascular network ensures efficient delivery of neurohypophyseal hormones to the systemic circulation, where they exert their physiological effects on target organs and tissues.

Relationship with Hypothalamic Nuclei:

The supraoptic and paraventricular nuclei of the hypothalamus are responsible for synthesizing the hormones oxytocin and vasopressin, respectively. These hormones are produced as larger precursor molecules (preprohormones) within the cell bodies of hypothalamic neurons. The preprohormones undergo post-translational processing within the endoplasmic reticulum and Golgi apparatus to form mature oxytocin and vasopressin. Once synthesized, these hormones are packaged into secretory vesicles and transported along axons to the nerve terminals in the posterior pituitary, where they are stored until release. The release of oxytocin and vasopressin from the neurohypophysis is tightly regulated by neuronal impulses originating in the hypothalamus in response to various physiological stimuli, including sensory inputs, osmotic changes, and stress.

5.2 Hormones Produced by Neurohypophysis:

Oxytocin

Oxytocin is a peptide hormone produced primarily in the hypothalamus, specifically in the paraventricular nucleus and, to a lesser extent, in the supraoptic nucleus. It is stored and released from the posterior pituitary gland, also known as the neurohypophysis. Oxytocin plays a crucial role in various physiological processes and behaviors, earning it the nickname "the love hormone" or "the bonding hormone."

Chemical Structure:

Oxytocin is a peptide hormone composed of nine amino acids. Its chemical structure consists of a cyclic six-membered ring with a disulfide bridge between two cysteine residues. This structure is crucial for its biological activity and stability.

1. Amino Acid Sequence: Oxytocin is composed of the following nine amino acids arranged in a specific sequence: Cysteine - Tyrosine - Isoleucine - Glutamine - Asparagine - Cysteine (forming a disulfide bridge with the first cysteine) - Proline - Leucine - Glycine

The amino acid residues form a cyclic structure, with the peptide bond between the first cysteine and glycine residues closing the ring. This cyclic structure enhances oxytocin's stability and resistance to enzymatic degradation. A disulfide bridge is formed between the two cysteine residues (at positions 1 and 6 in the amino acid sequence), creating a covalent bond between the sulfur atoms of the cysteine side chains. This disulfide bridge contributes to oxytocin's structural integrity and maintains its biological activity.

The chemical formula of oxytocin is $C_{43}H_{66}N_{12}O_{12}S_2$, reflecting the number and composition of its constituent atoms.

Synthesis and Secretions:

The synthesis and secretion of oxytocin involve several intricate steps, beginning in the hypothalamus and culminating in its release from the posterior pituitary gland. Here's a detailed explanation of the process:

1. Synthesis in the Hypothalamus:

- Oxytocin synthesis primarily occurs in the cell bodies of neurons located in the paraventricular nucleus (PVN) of the hypothalamus. These neurons contain the genetic instructions (oxytocin gene) necessary for oxytocin synthesis.

- The oxytocin gene is transcribed into messenger RNA (mRNA) in the cell nucleus. This mRNA serves as a template for protein synthesis, specifically the production of preprooxytocin.

- Preprooxytocin is a larger precursor molecule that undergoes post-translational modifications to form prooxytocin. These modifications include the removal of signal peptides and the addition of glycosylation.

- Prooxytocin is packaged into secretory vesicles within the cell's Golgi apparatus, preparing it for transport to the nerve terminals.

2. Transport to Posterior Pituitary:

- Once packaged into secretory vesicles, prooxytocin is transported along the axons of hypothalamic neurons to the nerve terminals located in the posterior pituitary gland.

- This transportation process involves microtubules and motor proteins that facilitate the movement of vesicles along the axonal cytoskeleton. It is a form of axonal transport known as anterograde transport.

3. Storage in the Posterior Pituitary:

- Upon reaching the nerve terminals in the posterior pituitary, the secretory vesicles containing oxytocin are stored until they receive signals for release.

- The nerve terminals in the posterior pituitary contain specialized machinery for the storage and release of oxytocin. These terminals are in close proximity to fenestrated capillaries, allowing for efficient hormone secretion into the bloodstream.

4. Release of Oxytocin:

- The release of oxytocin from the posterior pituitary is triggered by specific stimuli, such as mechanical or sensory signals associated with childbirth, breastfeeding, or social interactions.

- When these stimuli are detected, action potentials are generated in the oxytocin-secreting neurons of the hypothalamus. These action potentials propagate down the axons to the nerve terminals in the posterior pituitary.

- Upon reaching the nerve terminals, the action potentials trigger the opening of voltage-gated calcium channels, leading to an influx of calcium ions into the nerve terminals.

- The increase in intracellular calcium concentration triggers the fusion of the oxytocin-containing secretory vesicles with the plasma membrane, a process known as exocytosis. This results in the release of oxytocin into the bloodstream, where it can exert its physiological effects on target tissues and organs.

Functions:

- Uterine Contractions: One of the best-known functions of oxytocin is its role in uterine contractions during childbirth (parturition). Oxytocin stimulates the contraction of smooth muscle cells in the uterine wall, leading to labor and the eventual delivery of the baby.

- Milk Ejection (Let-Down Reflex): Oxytocin also plays a crucial role in facilitating milk ejection from the mammary glands during breastfeeding. When a baby suckles at the breast, sensory stimuli from the nipple trigger the release of oxytocin, causing the contraction of myoepithelial cells surrounding the alveoli and ducts of the mammary glands. This contraction propels milk from the alveoli into the ducts, allowing the baby to feed.

- Social Bonding and Affiliation: Oxytocin has been implicated in promoting social bonding, trust, and affiliation between individuals. Studies have shown that intranasal administration of oxytocin can increase feelings of trust and generosity towards others and enhance social behaviors, such as eye contact, empathy, and emotional bonding.

- Maternal Behaviors: Oxytocin is also involved in regulating maternal behaviors, such as nurturing, caregiving, and protective instincts towards offspring. Elevated levels of oxytocin have been observed in mothers during pregnancy, childbirth, and breastfeeding, facilitating the development of maternal bonding and attachment.

Clinical Applications:

Oxytocin has therapeutic potential in various clinical settings. It is used clinically to induce labor and augment uterine contractions during childbirth. Additionally, synthetic oxytocin analogs, such as Pitocin, are administered intravenously to manage postpartum hemorrhage and facilitate milk ejection during breastfeeding. Research into the therapeutic effects of oxytocin in conditions such as autism spectrum disorders, social anxiety, and depression is ongoing, although further studies are needed to elucidate its efficacy and safety in these contexts.

Vasopressin (Antidiuretic Hormone, ADH):

Vasopressin, also known as antidiuretic hormone (ADH), is another crucial hormone produced by the hypothalamus and released from the posterior pituitary gland. Vasopressin plays a vital role in regulating water balance and blood pressure, primarily through its effects on the kidneys and blood vessels.

Chemical Structure:

The chemical structure of vasopressin, also known as antidiuretic hormone (ADH), is composed of nine amino acids. It is a peptide hormone with the following chemical formula: $C_{46}H_{65}N_{13}O_{12}S_2$.

The structure of vasopressin consists of 00a cyclic six-membered ring formed by a disulfide bridge between two cysteine residues (Cys1 and Cys6), with a peptide bond linking the amino acids at positions 2 and 7. The side chains of the amino acids extend from the ring structure, forming the functional domains of the hormone.

The sequence of amino acids in vasopressin is as follows:

- Cys-Tyr-Phe-Gln-Asn-Cys-Pro-Arg-Gly

This sequence is essential for the biological activity of vasopressin, as it determines its ability to bind to specific receptors and initiate cellular responses in target tissues, such as the kidneys and blood vessels.

Synthesis and Secretion

Vasopressin, also known as antidiuretic hormone (ADH), is synthesized and secreted primarily by the hypothalamus, specifically in the supraoptic nucleus. The synthesis and secretion of vasopressin involve several intricate steps, which are crucial for its physiological functions in regulating water balance and blood pressure. Here's a detailed overview of the synthesis and secretion process:

1. Synthesis:

- Transcription: The synthesis of vasopressin begins with the transcription of the vasopressin gene into a larger precursor molecule called preprovasopressin. This process occurs in the cell bodies of neurons located in the supraoptic nucleus of the hypothalamus.

- Translation: The preprovasopressin mRNA is then translated into a preprohormone protein within the rough endoplasmic reticulum of the neuronal cell bodies. The preprohormone contains the entire sequence of vasopressin, along with a signal peptide that targets it for secretion.

- Post-Translational Modifications: After translation, the preprovasopressin undergoes several post-translational modifications, including cleavage and glycosylation, within the endoplasmic reticulum and Golgi apparatus. These modifications are essential for the maturation and processing of vasopressin into its active form.

- Formation of Provasopressin: The processed preprovasopressin is cleaved to produce provasopressin, which consists of the vasopressin peptide and a neurophysin carrier protein. Provasopressin is the precursor molecule for the mature vasopressin hormone.

2. Transport and Packaging:

- Axonal Transport: Once synthesized, provasopressin is packaged into secretory vesicles and transported along the axons of hypothalamic neurons to the nerve endings located in the posterior pituitary gland, also known as the neurohypophysis.

- Storage: Within the nerve endings of the posterior pituitary, provasopressin-containing secretory vesicles are stored in large quantities, awaiting appropriate signals for release into the bloodstream. These vesicles are localized near the capillary networks of the posterior pituitary, facilitating rapid release upon stimulation.

3. Secretion:

- Release Mechanism: The secretion of vasopressin from the posterior pituitary is regulated by neural and hormonal stimuli, primarily changes in plasma osmolality and blood volume. Increases in plasma osmolality or decreases in blood volume stimulate vasopressin release, while decreases in plasma osmolality or increases in blood volume inhibit vasopressin secretion.

- Action Potentials: When appropriate stimuli are detected, action potentials are generated in the hypothalamic neurons containing vasopressin. These action potentials propagate along the axons to the nerve endings in the posterior pituitary, leading to depolarization of the nerve terminals and the influx of calcium ions.

- Exocytosis: The increase in intracellular calcium triggers the fusion of vasopressin-containing secretory vesicles with the plasma membrane of the nerve endings. This fusion results in the exocytosis of vasopressin into the bloodstream, where it can exert its physiological effects on target organs, primarily the kidneys and blood vessels.

Clinical Applications:

Vasopressin and its synthetic analogs have clinical applications in various medical conditions, including:

- Diabetes Insipidus: Vasopressin or its synthetic analogs are used to treat central diabetes insipidus, a condition characterized by inadequate vasopressin secretion or action.

- Hemorrhagic Shock: Vasopressin may be used as a vasopressor agent to increase blood pressure and restore vascular tone in patients with severe hemorrhagic shock or hypotension.

- Cardiac Arrest: Vasopressin has been studied as an alternative vasopressor to epinephrine in the management of cardiac arrest, particularly in refractory cases.

5.3 Regulation of Neurohypophyseal Hormone Secretion:

The secretion of oxytocin and vasopressin (antidiuretic hormone, ADH) from the neurohypophysis (posterior pituitary) is tightly regulated by neural and non-neural inputs, ensuring precise control over their release in response to physiological stimuli. The regulation of neurohypophyseal hormone secretion involves complex mechanisms that integrate sensory, neural, and hormonal signals to maintain homeostasis.

Oxytocin Secretion Regulation:

Oxytocin secretion is primarily regulated by sensory stimuli associated with childbirth (parturition) and breastfeeding (lactation). The process involves a series of events that trigger neuronal signals leading to oxytocin release from the hypothalamus. Here's a detailed explanation of the regulation of oxytocin secretion:

1. Childbirth (Parturition):

- During labor and delivery, rhythmic contractions of the uterine muscles occur to facilitate the expulsion of the fetus.

- Stretching of the uterine cervix and vagina, particularly during the later stages of labor, activates sensory receptors known as mechanoreceptors.

- These mechanoreceptors detect the stretching of the uterine walls and transmit neuronal impulses to the brain, specifically to the hypothalamus.

- Within the hypothalamus, oxytocin-producing neurons located in the paraventricular nucleus receive these neuronal signals.

- The increased neuronal activity in response to uterine stretching leads to enhanced synthesis and release of oxytocin from the nerve terminals in the posterior pituitary gland.

- Oxytocin then enters the bloodstream and binds to oxytocin receptors on the smooth muscle cells of the uterus, promoting further uterine contractions.

- This positive feedback loop between uterine stretching, oxytocin release, and uterine contractions helps to progress labor and facilitate childbirth.

2. Breastfeeding (Lactation):

- During breastfeeding, the suckling action of the infant on the mother's nipple and areola stimulates sensory nerve endings in the breast.

- These sensory nerves transmit signals to the brain, particularly to the hypothalamus, signaling the initiation of breastfeeding.

- The hypothalamus responds to the sensory input by increasing neuronal activity in oxytocin-producing neurons within the paraventricular nucleus.

- This heightened neuronal activity leads to the synthesis and release of oxytocin from the nerve terminals in the posterior pituitary gland.

- Oxytocin released into the bloodstream reaches the mammary glands, where it binds to oxytocin receptors on myoepithelial cells surrounding the alveoli (milk-producing cells).

- Oxytocin binding to its receptors triggers the contraction of myoepithelial cells, causing the expulsion of milk from the alveoli into the lactiferous ducts.

- This milk ejection reflex, also known as the let-down reflex, allows milk to flow from the breast and be available for the infant's feeding.

In summary, oxytocin secretion during childbirth and breastfeeding is regulated by sensory stimuli that activate oxytocin-producing neurons in the hypothalamus.

These stimuli initiate a cascade of events leading to oxytocin release from the posterior pituitary gland, which in turn facilitates uterine contractions during labor and promotes milk ejection during breastfeeding, essential for successful childbirth and lactation.

Vasopressin (Antidiuretic Hormone, ADH) Secretion Regulation:

Vasopressin secretion is tightly regulated by various physiological factors to maintain water balance and blood pressure within narrow limits. The regulation of ADH secretion involves intricate mechanisms that integrate sensory, neural, and hormonal signals originating from the central nervous system and peripheral tissues.

1. Osmoreceptor Regulation:

- Osmoreceptors located in the hypothalamus, particularly the supraoptic and paraventricular nuclei, are specialized neurons that sense changes in plasma osmolality (osmotic pressure).

- An increase in plasma osmolality, indicating dehydration or increased solute concentration, stimulates osmoreceptor activation.

- Activated osmoreceptors signal the hypothalamus to increase vasopressin synthesis and release from the neurohypophysis (posterior pituitary).

- Vasopressin acts on the kidneys to enhance water reabsorption in the renal collecting ducts, reducing urine volume and increasing urine osmolality, thereby conserving body fluids and restoring plasma osmolality to normal levels.

- Conversely, a decrease in plasma osmolality inhibits osmoreceptor activity and suppresses vasopressin secretion, allowing increased water excretion in the urine to reduce fluid retention and maintain osmotic balance.

2. Baroreceptor Regulation:

- Baroreceptors are specialized stretch receptors located in blood vessels and the heart, particularly in the carotid sinus and aortic arch.

- Baroreceptors monitor changes in blood pressure and blood volume, detecting alterations in vascular filling and arterial pressure.

- Decreased blood volume or blood pressure, as occurs during dehydration, hemorrhage, or hypovolemia, stimulates baroreceptor activation.

- Activated baroreceptors transmit signals to the hypothalamus and brainstem nuclei involved in vasopressin regulation.

- The hypothalamus responds by increasing vasopressin secretion, leading to vasoconstriction and water reabsorption in the kidneys to restore blood pressure and volume.

3. Other Factors Influencing Vasopressin Secretion:

- Pain, stress, nausea, and certain medications can also modulate vasopressin secretion via neural and hormonal pathways.

- Factors such as angiotensin II, endothelin, and prostaglandins can stimulate vasopressin release indirectly by altering vascular tone and renal perfusion.

- Alcohol and caffeine consumption can inhibit vasopressin secretion, leading to increased urine production and potential dehydration.

In summary, the regulation of vasopressin secretion is governed by a sophisticated interplay of osmoreceptor and baroreceptor inputs, as well as various hormonal and neural factors, to maintain water balance, blood pressure, and osmotic homeostasis. Dysregulation of ADH secretion can lead to disorders such as diabetes insipidus (characterized by excessive urine production and thirst) or syndrome of inappropriate antidiuretic hormone secretion (SIADH, characterized by excessive water retention and dilutional hyponatremia). Understanding the mechanisms underlying vasopressin regulation is essential for managing fluid and electrolyte imbalances and treating associated disorders effectively.

5.4 Conclusion

In conclusion, the neurohypophyseal system, or posterior pituitary, is a key component of the endocrine system responsible for the synthesis and secretion of oxytocin and vasopressin. These hormones play diverse and critical roles in regulating physiological processes such as water balance, reproduction, and social behaviors.

Oxytocin, known as the "love hormone" or "bonding hormone," facilitates uterine contractions during childbirth, promotes milk ejection during breastfeeding, and fosters social bonding and trust between individuals. Vasopressin, also known as antidiuretic hormone (ADH), regulates water balance by increasing water reabsorption in the kidneys, thereby reducing urine output and conserving body fluids. Additionally, vasopressin plays a role in controlling blood pressure and vascular tone through its vasoconstrictor effects.

The synthesis, secretion, functions, and regulation of oxytocin and vasopressin are tightly controlled by neural and non-neural inputs acting on hypothalamic neurons. Sensory stimuli associated with childbirth, breastfeeding, plasma osmolality, and blood volume regulate the release of these hormones to maintain homeostasis.

Understanding the intricate mechanisms underlying the neurohypophyseal system provides insights into its physiological significance and clinical implications in various conditions, including water balance disorders, reproductive disorders, and social dysfunction.

Continued research in neuroendocrinology will further elucidate the complexities of the neurohypophyseal system and its potential therapeutic applications in managing endocrine-related disorders and enhancing human health and well-being.

Case Studies

Case Study 1: Diabetes Insipidus

Patient Profile:

- Name: Sarah Thompson

- Age: 28 years

- Sex: Female

- Occupation: Teacher

- Medical History: No significant medical history

- Family History: No known endocrine disorders

Presentation:

Sarah presents to her primary care physician with complaints of excessive thirst and urination over the past several weeks. She reports drinking up to 10 liters of water daily and waking up multiple times during the night to urinate. She feels fatigued and has experienced weight loss despite maintaining her usual diet.

Physical Examination:

- Vital Signs: BP: 110/70 mmHg, HR: 80 bpm, Temp: 36.6°C

- General Appearance: Thin, appears dehydrated

- Skin and Mucous Membranes: Dry mucous membranes, skin turgor decreased

Laboratory Tests:

- Serum Sodium: Elevated

- Serum Osmolality: Elevated

- Urine Osmolality: Low

- Urine Specific Gravity: Low

Discussion:

Sarah's symptoms and laboratory findings suggest diabetes insipidus, a condition characterized by insufficient production or action of antidiuretic hormone (ADH), leading to excessive excretion of dilute urine and subsequent dehydration and hypernatremia.

Questions:

1. Explain the role of ADH in water homeostasis.

2. Differentiate between central and nephrogenic diabetes insipidus.

3. What are the expected changes in serum and urine osmolality in a patient with diabetes insipidus?

4. Describe the diagnostic tests used to differentiate between central and nephrogenic diabetes insipidus.

Case Study 2: Syndrome of Inappropriate Antidiuretic Hormone Secretion (SIADH)

Patient Profile:

- Name: Michael Johnson

- Age: 65 years

- Sex: Male

- Occupation: Retired

- Medical History: Small cell lung carcinoma

- Family History: No significant family history

Presentation:

Michael presents to the emergency department with confusion, headache, and muscle cramps. His wife reports that he has been increasingly lethargic and has had a poor appetite. He has not had significant changes in fluid intake but seems to be retaining water.

Physical Examination:

- Vital Signs: BP: 140/85 mmHg, HR: 75 bpm, Temp: 37.0°C

- General Appearance: Confused, appears euvolemic

- Neurological Examination: No focal deficits but is disoriented

Laboratory Tests:

- Serum Sodium: Low

- Serum Osmolality: Low

- Urine Osmolality: High

- Urine Sodium: High

Discussion:

Michael's clinical presentation and laboratory results suggest SIADH, a condition where excessive release of ADH leads to water retention, hyponatremia, and low serum osmolality. SIADH is often associated with malignancies, such as small cell lung carcinoma.

Questions:

1. Explain the pathophysiology of SIADH.

2. What are the diagnostic criteria for SIADH?

3. Describe the clinical manifestations of SIADH.

4. How is SIADH managed and treated in clinical practice?

Practice Questions for Self-Assessment

Multiple Choice Questions

1. Which hormone is primarily released by the posterior pituitary gland?

   a) Prolactin

   b) Thyroid-stimulating hormone (TSH)

   c) Antidiuretic hormone (ADH)

   d) Adrenocorticotropic hormone (ACTH)

2. The primary function of oxytocin is:

   a) Regulation of blood glucose levels

   b) Stimulation of milk ejection during lactation

   c) Control of metabolic rate

d) Regulation of calcium homeostasis

3. Which of the following is a common cause of central diabetes insipidus?

   a) Kidney disease

   b) Autoimmune thyroiditis

   c) Pituitary tumor

   d) Excessive fluid intake

4. In SIADH, which of the following laboratory findings is typically observed?

   a) High serum sodium

   b) Low urine osmolality

   c) High serum osmolality

   d) Low serum sodium

5. Which hormone acts on the kidneys to promote water reabsorption?

   a) Aldosterone

   b) Insulin

   c) ADH

   d) Parathyroid hormone (PTH)

Short Answer Questions

1. Describe the synthesis and release process of ADH.

2. Explain the role of oxytocin during childbirth.

3. Discuss how ADH contributes to the regulation of blood pressure.

4. What are the physiological effects of a deficiency in ADH?

5. Describe the mechanisms by which oxytocin facilitates social bonding.

True or False Questions

1. ADH is also known as vasopressin. (True/False)

2. Oxytocin is involved in the regulation of blood calcium levels. (True/False)

3. The neurohypophysis is another term for the anterior pituitary gland. (True/False)

4. SIADH can result in hyponatremia. (True/False)

5. ADH increases the permeability of the kidney's collecting ducts to water. (True/False)

Answers

Case Study 1

1. Role of ADH in Water Homeostasis:

- ADH, also known as vasopressin, is released from the posterior pituitary in response to increased plasma osmolality or decreased blood volume. It acts on the kidneys to increase water reabsorption, reducing urine output and concentrating the urine. This helps maintain plasma osmolality and blood volume within normal ranges.

2. Central vs. Nephrogenic Diabetes Insipidus:

- Central diabetes insipidus results from a deficiency in ADH production or secretion, often due to damage to the hypothalamus or pituitary gland. Nephrogenic diabetes insipidus occurs when the kidneys do not respond properly to ADH, despite normal or elevated levels of the hormone. This can be due to genetic defects, certain medications, or kidney disease.

3. Serum and Urine Osmolality in Diabetes Insipidus:

- In diabetes insipidus, serum osmolality is elevated due to excessive loss of free water. Urine osmolality is low because the kidneys are unable to concentrate urine in the absence or ineffectiveness of ADH. This results in the excretion of large volumes of dilute urine.

4. Diagnostic Tests for Diabetes Insipidus:

- The water deprivation test helps differentiate between central and nephrogenic diabetes insipidus. In central DI, urine osmolality increases significantly after administration of synthetic ADH (desmopressin), indicating the kidneys can respond to the hormone. In nephrogenic DI, there is little or no increase in urine osmolality, indicating the kidneys do not respond to ADH.

Case Study 2

1. Pathophysiology of SIADH:

- SIADH involves excessive release of ADH, leading to water retention and dilutional hyponatremia. This results in low serum osmolality, concentrated urine, and increased urine sodium. The excess water retention causes a relative reduction in sodium concentration, leading to symptoms of hyponatremia.

2. Diagnostic Criteria for SIADH:

- The diagnosis of SIADH includes low serum osmolality, low serum sodium, high urine osmolality, and high urine sodium in the absence of hypovolemia, edema, or other causes of hyponatremia. Exclusion of other potential causes of hyponatremia, such as renal, adrenal, or thyroid dysfunction, is also necessary.

3. Clinical Manifestations of SIADH:

- Symptoms of SIADH include headache, confusion, lethargy, muscle cramps, nausea, and vomiting. Severe hyponatremia can lead to cerebral edema, seizures, and coma. Patients often appear euvolemic, without signs of significant fluid overload or dehydration.

4. Management and Treatment of SIADH:

- Treatment involves addressing the underlying cause (e.g., malignancy), restricting fluid intake, and correcting hyponatremia. In severe cases, hypertonic saline may be administered cautiously to raise serum sodium levels. Medications such as demeclocycline or vasopressin receptor antagonists (vaptans) may be used to reduce ADH activity.

Multiple Choice Questions

1. c) Antidiuretic hormone (ADH)

2. b) Stimulation of milk ejection during lactation

3. c) Pituitary tumor

4. d) Low serum sodium

5. c) ADH

Short Answer Questions

1. Synthesis and Release of ADH:

- ADH is synthesized in the hypothalamus and stored in the posterior pituitary gland. It is released into the bloodstream in response to increased plasma osmolality or decreased blood volume. ADH then acts on the kidneys to promote water reabsorption, concentrating the urine and maintaining fluid balance.

2. Role of Oxytocin During Childbirth:

- Oxytocin is released from the posterior pituitary during childbirth. It stimulates uterine contractions, helping to dilate the cervix and facilitate labor. It also promotes milk ejection during breastfeeding by causing contraction of myoepithelial cells around the mammary glands.

3. ADH and Blood Pressure Regulation:

- ADH increases water reabsorption in the kidneys, which helps maintain blood volume and, consequently, blood pressure. Additionally, at high concentrations, ADH can cause vasoconstriction, further contributing to blood pressure regulation.

4. Effects of ADH Deficiency:

- A deficiency in ADH leads to diabetes insipidus, characterized by excessive urination (polyuria) and excessive thirst (polydipsia). The inability to concentrate urine results in the excretion of large volumes of dilute urine, dehydration, and potential electrolyte imbalances.

5. Oxytocin and Social Bonding:

- Oxytocin is often referred to as the "love hormone" because it plays a role in social bonding, maternal behaviors, and trust. It enhances bonding between mother and infant during breastfeeding and is involved in forming social relationships and emotional connections.

True or False Questions

1. True

2. False

3. False

4. True

5. True

Bibliography

1. Kandel, E. R., Schwartz, J. H., & Jessell, T. M. (2000). Principles of Neural Science (4th ed.). McGraw-Hill.

   - This comprehensive textbook provides in-depth coverage of the neural control of the endocrine system, including the role of the hypothalamus and posterior pituitary hormones.

2. Golan, D. E., Tashjian, A. H., Armstrong, E. J., & Galanter, J. M. (2017). Principles of Pharmacology: The Pathophysiologic Basis of Drug Therapy (4th ed.). Wolters Kluwer.

   - Offers detailed insights into the pharmacological aspects and physiological mechanisms of neurohypophyseal hormones, particularly oxytocin and vasopressin.

3. Guyton, A. C., & Hall, J. E. (2016). Guyton and Hall Textbook of Medical Physiology (13th ed.). Elsevier.

- An essential resource for understanding the physiological processes of the posterior pituitary and the regulation of its hormone secretion.

4. Sadler, T. W. (2018). Langman's Medical Embryology (14th ed.). Lippincott Williams & Wilkins.

   - Provides detailed information on the embryological development of the hypothalamus and posterior pituitary, enhancing understanding of their physiological functions.

5. Boron, W. F., & Boulpaep, E. L. (2016). Medical Physiology (3rd ed.). Elsevier.

   - A comprehensive textbook that covers the physiological principles and regulatory mechanisms of the neurohypophyseal system.

6. Rang, H. P., Dale, M. M., Ritter, J. M., Flower, R. J., & Henderson, G. (2016). Rang and Dale's Pharmacology (8th ed.). Elsevier.

   - Provides pharmacological perspectives on the actions and therapeutic applications of vasopressin and oxytocin, highlighting their clinical significance.

7. Goodman, H. M. (2009). Basic Medical Endocrinology (4th ed.). Academic Press.

   - Focuses on the fundamental aspects of endocrine physiology, including the role of the posterior pituitary hormones in maintaining homeostasis.

8. Hadley, M. E., & Levine, J. E. (2007). Endocrinology (6th ed.). Pearson.

   - This textbook offers a detailed exploration of the endocrine system, emphasizing the functional aspects of the neurohypophyseal hormones.

9. Sherwood, L. (2015). Human Physiology: From Cells to Systems (9th ed.). Cengage Learning.

   - Covers the integrated functions of the neurohypophyseal system within the broader context of human physiology.

10. Fitzgerald, P. A. (2018). Handbook of Clinical Neuroendocrinology (2nd ed.). Wiley-Blackwell.

    - This handbook provides clinical insights and case studies on disorders related to the neurohypophyseal hormones, offering a bridge between physiology and clinical practice.

Chapter 6

Physiology of Growth and Growth Factors

Growth is a fundamental process in biology, essential for the development, maintenance, and repair of tissues and organs throughout the lifespan. In this chapter, we explore the intricate mechanisms underlying growth regulation, focusing on the role of growth hormone and growth factors in orchestrating cellular proliferation, differentiation, and tissue growth.

6.1 Growth Hormone: Structure and Synthesis

Growth hormone (GH), also known as somatotropin, is a peptide hormone composed of 191 amino acids. Its primary structure consists of a single polypeptide chain with two disulfide bridges. This compact structure is essential for its stability and biological activity.

Structure of Growth Hormone:

The structure of growth hormone (GH), also known as somatotropin, is essential for its stability, secretion, and biological activity. GH is a peptide hormone composed of 191 amino acids arranged in a specific sequence. Let's explore the structure of GH in detail:

Primary Structure:

- GH is a single polypeptide chain consisting of 191 amino acids.

- The primary structure of GH is determined by the sequence of amino acids encoded by the GH gene (GH1).

- This sequence is crucial for the proper folding and function of the hormone.

Secondary Structure:

- The secondary structure of GH is predominantly alpha-helical.

- Alpha-helices are formed when the polypeptide chain twists into a helical shape stabilized by hydrogen bonds between amino acids.

- GH contains four alpha-helices, labeled helices A, B, C, and D.

Tertiary Structure:

- The tertiary structure of GH refers to the three-dimensional arrangement of the alpha-helices and other structural elements.

- GH adopts a compact, globular conformation stabilized by intramolecular interactions, including hydrogen bonds and disulfide bridges.

- The tertiary structure is essential for maintaining the stability and biological activity of GH.

Disulfide Bridges:

- Disulfide bridges are covalent bonds formed between two cysteine residues through oxidation of their sulfur atoms.

- GH contains two disulfide bridges that contribute to its structural integrity.

- These disulfide bridges help stabilize the tertiary structure of GH and protect it from denaturation.

Functional Domains:

- The structure of GH includes functional domains responsible for hormone-receptor interactions and biological activity.

- Helices A and B form the primary hormone-binding site, where GH interacts with its receptor on target cells.

- Other regions of GH, including helices C and D, may also play a role in receptor binding and signaling.

Post-Translational Modifications:

- After synthesis, GH undergoes post-translational modifications that further shape its structure and function.

- These modifications may include glycosylation, phosphorylation, and proteolytic cleavage.

- Post-translational modifications can affect the stability, secretion, and activity of GH.

Synthesis of Growth Hormone:

The synthesis of Growth Hormone (GH) is a multistep process that begins with the transcription of the GH gene in response to regulatory signals. This process occurs primarily in the somatotropic cells located in the anterior pituitary gland. Here's a detailed breakdown of the synthesis of GH:

1. Gene Transcription:

- The GH gene, also known as GH1, is located on chromosome 17 in humans. It consists of multiple exons and introns that encode the GH precursor protein, preproghrelin.

- Transcription of the GH gene is regulated by hypothalamic hormones, primarily Growth Hormone-Releasing Hormone (GHRH) and Somatostatin (also known as Growth Hormone-Inhibiting Hormone, GHIH).

- GHRH stimulates GH gene transcription, leading to increased synthesis of preproghrelin mRNA.

- Conversely, Somatostatin inhibits GH gene transcription, resulting in decreased synthesis of preproghrelin mRNA.

- The transcriptional regulation of the GH gene by GHRH and Somatostatin ensures tight control over GH synthesis and secretion in response to physiological stimuli.

2. Translation and Post-Translational Modification:

- The preproghrelin mRNA is transcribed in the nucleus and undergoes translation on ribosomes bound to the rough endoplasmic reticulum (ER).

- The nascent preproghrelin polypeptide consists of a signal peptide sequence at the N-terminus, which targets it for translocation into the ER lumen.

- As preproghrelin is translocated into the ER, the signal peptide is cleaved off, resulting in the formation of proghrelin.

- Proghrelin undergoes further post-translational modifications in the ER and Golgi apparatus, including glycosylation and proteolytic processing, to generate mature GH.

- These post-translational modifications are essential for the proper folding, stability, and biological activity of GH.

3. Packaging and Secretion:

- Mature GH molecules are packaged into secretory vesicles within the somatotropic cells.

- These secretory vesicles accumulate near the plasma membrane, awaiting signals for exocytosis and secretion.

- GH secretion is pulsatile, with episodes of secretion occurring throughout the day in response to various physiological stimuli such as sleep, exercise, stress, and nutritional status.

- Upon stimulation, the secretory vesicles fuse with the plasma membrane, releasing GH into the bloodstream.

4. Regulation of Secretion:

- The secretion of GH is tightly regulated by a complex interplay of hypothalamic, peripheral, and feedback mechanisms.

- Hypothalamic hormones, including GHRH and Somatostatin, act on somatotropic cells to stimulate or inhibit GH secretion, respectively.

- Peripheral factors such as blood glucose levels, amino acids, and stress hormones also modulate GH secretion through direct and indirect mechanisms.

6.2 Mechanisms of Action of Growth Hormone:

Growth hormone (GH) exerts its effects on target tissues through both direct and indirect mechanisms, orchestrating a wide array of physiological processes crucial for growth, development, and metabolism. Understanding the intricate mechanisms underlying GH action is essential for comprehending its diverse biological effects.

Direct Effects of Growth Hormone:

GH binds to specific cell surface receptors, known as growth hormone receptors (GHRs), present on target cells throughout the body. These receptors belong to the cytokine receptor superfamily and are primarily located on hepatocytes, adipocytes, myocytes, chondrocytes, and osteoblasts.

Upon binding to GHRs, GH triggers a cascade of intracellular signaling events that culminate in various cellular responses:

1. Activation of Janus kinase (JAK)-signal transducer and activator of transcription (STAT) pathway: GH binding induces conformational changes in GHRs, leading to the activation of associated JAK kinases (JAK2). Activated JAK2 phosphorylates tyrosine residues on the GHR, creating docking sites for STAT proteins. Phosphorylated STAT proteins translocate to the nucleus, where they regulate gene transcription, leading to the expression of genes involved in cell growth, proliferation, and differentiation.

2. Activation of mitogen-activated protein kinase (MAPK) pathway: GH stimulation also activates the MAPK pathway, involving the sequential activation of Ras, Raf, MEK, and ERK kinases. ERK activation leads to the phosphorylation of transcription factors and other cytoplasmic proteins, regulating gene expression and cellular processes such as cell cycle progression, survival, and differentiation.

3. Regulation of gene expression: GH-mediated signaling pathways modulate the expression of a wide range of genes involved in cell growth, metabolism, and differentiation. These genes encode proteins involved in cell cycle regulation (cyclins, cyclin-dependent kinases), protein synthesis (ribosomal proteins, translation factors), and cell survival (Bcl-2 family proteins).

Indirect Effects of Growth Hormone via Insulin-like Growth Factor 1 (IGF-1):

GH stimulates the production of insulin-like growth factor 1 (IGF-1), primarily in the liver but also in other tissues such as muscle, bone, and adipose tissue. IGF-1, also known as somatomedin C, acts as a key mediator of GH's growth-promoting effects.

1. Hepatic synthesis of IGF-1: GH stimulates the transcription and translation of IGF-1 mRNA in hepatocytes, leading to increased synthesis and secretion of IGF-1 into the bloodstream. Hepatic IGF-1 production is the primary source of circulating IGF-1, which exerts endocrine effects on distant target tissues.

2. Local production of IGF-1: In addition to its endocrine actions, GH stimulates the production of IGF-1 in target tissues such as muscle, bone, and cartilage. Locally produced IGF-1 acts in a paracrine or autocrine manner to promote tissue growth, repair, and remodeling.

3. IGF-1 signaling pathways: IGF-1 binds to specific cell surface receptors, known as insulin-like growth factor 1 receptors (IGF-1Rs), initiating signaling cascades similar to those activated by insulin receptors. IGF-1R signaling regulates cell growth, proliferation, survival, and metabolism through activation of PI3K-Akt and MAPK pathways.

Integration of Direct and Indirect Effects:

The direct and indirect effects of GH synergistically regulate cellular growth, proliferation, and differentiation in various target tissues. While the direct effects of GH primarily influence immediate cellular responses, such as protein synthesis and cell growth, the indirect effects mediated by IGF-1 contribute to long-term growth and tissue remodeling processes.

Moreover, the interplay between GH and IGF-1 signaling pathways ensures tight regulation of growth processes, allowing for adaptation to changing physiological conditions and environmental cues. Dysregulation of GH signaling, either through excess or deficiency, can lead to growth disorders such as gigantism, dwarfism, and acromegaly, highlighting the importance of maintaining proper GH-IGF-1 axis function for normal growth and development.

6.3 Regulation of Growth Hormone Secretion

The secretion of growth hormone (GH), a pivotal regulator of growth and metabolism, is intricately governed by a multifaceted interplay of neural, hormonal, and metabolic factors. This dynamic regulation ensures that GH release is finely tuned to meet the body's physiological demands, particularly during periods of growth, stress, and metabolic challenges.

Neural Regulation:

The hypothalamus, a crucial neuroendocrine center in the brain, plays a central role in orchestrating the secretion of GH. Within the hypothalamus, specialized neurons produce and release two key regulatory peptides: growth hormone-releasing hormone (GHRH) and somatostatin (also known as growth hormone-inhibiting hormone, GHIH).

GHRH acts as a stimulatory signal for GH synthesis and release, promoting the activity of somatotroph cells in the anterior pituitary gland. It is secreted in response to various stimuli, including circadian rhythms, sleep-wake cycles, stressors, and nutritional status. During periods of fasting or low blood glucose levels, GHRH secretion is augmented, stimulating GH release and facilitating the mobilization of stored energy sources.

Conversely, somatostatin acts as an inhibitory signal for GH secretion, exerting its effects by binding to receptors on somatotroph cells in the anterior pituitary gland. Somatostatin inhibits the synthesis and release of GH in response to elevated blood glucose levels, high circulating GH concentrations, and other physiological stressors. By fine-tuning the balance between GHRH and somatostatin signaling, the hypothalamus maintains GH secretion within a physiologically appropriate range, preventing excessive or inadequate GH release.

Hormonal Regulation:

In addition to neural inputs, GH secretion is modulated by various hormonal signals originating from peripheral tissues and organs. These hormonal signals integrate information about metabolic status, nutrient availability, and physiological demands to regulate GH release accordingly.

Changes in blood glucose levels play a crucial role in modulating GH secretion. Hypoglycemia, or low blood glucose levels, triggers an increase in GH release through several mechanisms. Specialized glucose-sensing neurons in the hypothalamus detect decreases in blood glucose levels and respond by enhancing GHRH secretion while suppressing somatostatin release. Additionally, hypoglycemia directly stimulates GH secretion from somatotroph cells in the anterior pituitary gland, promoting the mobilization of glucose and fatty acids from storage depots.

Amino acids, particularly arginine and leucine, have been shown to stimulate GH secretion when administered orally or intravenously. These amino acids act directly on the hypothalamus and pituitary gland to enhance GHRH release and inhibit somatostatin secretion, leading to increased GH release. The stimulatory effects of amino acids on GH secretion are mediated by activation of amino acid-sensing receptors and subsequent intracellular signaling pathways within the hypothalamus and pituitary gland.

Stress hormones, such as cortisol and catecholamines (epinephrine and norepinephrine), also play a role in regulating GH secretion. Stressful situations, such as physical exertion, trauma, or emotional stress, activate the hypothalamic-pituitary-adrenal (HPA) axis, leading to increased GH release. Cortisol and catecholamines enhance GH secretion by stimulating GHRH release and suppressing somatostatin secretion, thereby mobilizing energy reserves and supporting the body's response to acute stressors.

Metabolic Regulation:

GH secretion is further influenced by metabolic signals arising from peripheral tissues and organs, reflecting the body's energy balance and nutritional status. Prolonged fasting or starvation is associated with increased GH secretion as a compensatory mechanism to maintain blood glucose levels and provide energy substrates for vital organs. During fasting, decreased insulin and increased glucagon levels promote lipolysis and gluconeogenesis, leading to increased release of fatty acids and glucose into the bloodstream. GH plays a critical role in promoting lipolysis and sparing glucose utilization by peripheral tissues, thereby conserving glucose for essential metabolic functions in the brain and red blood cells.

Conversely, obesity and insulin resistance are associated with blunted GH secretion and reduced sensitivity of target tissues to GH action, a phenomenon known as GH resistance. Hyperinsulinemia and elevated circulating levels of free fatty acids in obese individuals contribute to impaired GH secretion and signaling pathways. The pathophysiology of GH resistance in obesity is complex and multifactorial, involving interactions between adipose tissue-derived hormones, proinflammatory cytokines, and insulin signaling pathways.

6.4 Growth Factors

Insulin-like Growth Factors (IGFs):

Insulin-like Growth Factors (IGFs) are a family of peptide hormones that play crucial roles in mediating the effects of growth hormone (GH) on cellular growth, proliferation, and metabolism. There are two main members of the IGF family: IGF-1 and IGF-2.

Insulin-like Growth Factor 1 (IGF-1:

Insulin-like Growth Factor 1 (IGF-1), also known as somatomedin C, is a peptide hormone that plays a pivotal role in mediating the effects of growth hormone (GH) on growth, development, and metabolism. Here's a detailed exploration of IGF-1:

1. Synthesis and Secretion:

- IGF-1 is primarily synthesized and secreted by hepatocytes in the liver, under the stimulation of GH. It is also produced locally in various tissues, including skeletal muscle, bone, and adipose tissue.

- GH acts on the liver to stimulate the synthesis of IGF-1. Upon binding to its receptor on hepatocytes, GH activates signaling pathways that lead to the transcription and translation of the IGF-1 gene, resulting in the production and secretion of IGF-1 into the bloodstream.

2. Structure:

- IGF-1 is a single-chain polypeptide consisting of 70 amino acids. It shares structural homology with insulin, which is why it is termed "insulin-like."

- Despite its structural similarity to insulin, IGF-1 binds to its own specific cell surface receptor, the IGF-1 receptor (IGF-1R), initiating distinct intracellular signaling cascades.

3. Functions:

- Cellular Growth and Proliferation: IGF-1 exerts potent mitogenic effects on a wide range of cell types, including osteoblasts, chondrocytes, myocytes, and fibroblasts. It promotes cellular proliferation, differentiation, and hypertrophy, contributing to tissue growth and repair.

- Anabolic Effects: IGF-1 stimulates protein synthesis and inhibits protein degradation in skeletal muscle and other tissues. It enhances the incorporation of amino acids into proteins, leading to increased muscle mass and lean body mass.

- Metabolic Effects: IGF-1 shares metabolic actions with insulin, albeit to a lesser extent. It enhances glucose uptake and utilization in peripheral tissues, similar to insulin, and promotes glycogen synthesis and lipogenesis. Additionally, IGF-1 inhibits hepatic gluconeogenesis, contributing to the regulation of blood glucose levels.

4. Regulation:

- The synthesis and secretion of IGF-1 are primarily regulated by GH. GH secretion is pulsatile, with peaks occurring primarily during sleep and in response to various stimuli such as exercise, stress, and fasting.

- Growth hormone-releasing hormone (GHRH) and somatostatin (GHIH), produced by the hypothalamus, regulate GH secretion indirectly, thereby influencing IGF-1 production.

- Nutritional status, insulin levels, and other growth factors also modulate IGF-1 synthesis and secretion.

5. Clinical Implications:

- Deficiencies or dysregulation of IGF-1 signaling are associated with various pathological conditions:

- Laron syndrome: A rare genetic disorder characterized by IGF-1 resistance, resulting in severe growth retardation and dwarfism.

- Acromegaly: Excess GH secretion in adulthood leads to overproduction of IGF-1, resulting in abnormal growth of tissues, particularly in the hands, feet, and face.

- Insulin resistance: Impaired IGF-1 signaling has been implicated in insulin resistance and metabolic disorders such as type 2 diabetes mellitus and obesity.

- Cancer: Dysregulated IGF-1 signaling is associated with the development and progression of various cancers, including breast, prostate, and colorectal cancer, where IGF-1 acts as a potent mitogen promoting tumor cell proliferation.

Insulin-like Growth Factor 2 (IGF-2):

IGF-2 is a peptide hormone that belongs to the insulin-like growth factor family, alongside IGF-1. It plays a pivotal role in fetal growth and development, particularly during embryogenesis and organogenesis. Here's a detailed exploration of IGF-2:

1. Synthesis and Secretion:

- IGF-2 is primarily synthesized during fetal development, with its expression tightly regulated during embryogenesis.

- The production of IGF-2 occurs predominantly in fetal tissues, including the liver, placenta, and other embryonic tissues.

- Unlike IGF-1, which is mainly regulated by growth hormone (GH), the synthesis and secretion of IGF-2 are influenced by complex mechanisms involving genomic imprinting and epigenetic regulation.

- IGF-2 is subject to genomic imprinting, where the expression of the gene is determined by parental origin. The paternal allele is typically expressed, while the maternal allele is silenced in most tissues.

2. Functions:

- Fetal Growth and Development: IGF-2 is a potent mitogen and plays a crucial role in stimulating cellular proliferation and differentiation during fetal development. It promotes the growth and development of various organs and tissues, including the liver, skeletal muscle, and central nervous system.

- Placental Function: IGF-2 is also involved in regulating placental growth and function, facilitating nutrient and oxygen exchange between the mother and fetus.

- Organogenesis: During embryogenesis, IGF-2 is essential for the patterning and differentiation of various tissues and organs. It influences processes such as limb development, organ morphogenesis, and neural tube formation.

- Autocrine and Paracrine Signaling: IGF-2 acts via autocrine and paracrine mechanisms, exerting its effects on nearby cells to coordinate tissue growth and differentiation.

3. Regulation:

- The expression of IGF-2 is tightly regulated at the transcriptional, post-transcriptional, and epigenetic levels.

- Imprinted gene control regions, such as differentially methylated regions (DMRs), play a crucial role in regulating IGF-2 expression by controlling allele-specific gene expression.

- Growth factors, hormones, and environmental cues also modulate IGF-2 expression during development and in response to physiological stimuli.

4. Clinical Implications:

- Dysregulation of IGF-2 expression and signaling is associated with various developmental disorders and cancers.

- Beckwith-Wiedemann syndrome (BWS), characterized by overgrowth and developmental abnormalities, is often associated with dysregulation of IGF-2 expression due to alterations in genomic imprinting.

- Aberrant expression of IGF-2 has been observed in various cancers, including hepatocellular carcinoma, colorectal cancer, and Wilms tumor, where it promotes tumor cell proliferation and survival.

Epidermal Growth Factors (EGFs):

Epidermal growth factors (EGFs) are a family of polypeptide growth factors that play crucial roles in regulating cell proliferation, differentiation, and tissue repair, particularly in the skin and other epithelial tissues. Discovered by Stanley Cohen in the 1960s, EGF was the first member of this family to be identified and characterized.

Key aspects of EGFs include:

1. Structure and Synthesis: EGFs are small polypeptides typically composed of 53 to 84 amino acids. The prototypical EGF is a 53-amino acid peptide derived from a larger precursor protein. EGFs are produced by various cell types, including keratinocytes, fibroblasts, and macrophages, and are secreted into the extracellular environment.

2. Receptor Interaction: EGF exerts its biological effects by binding to the EGF receptor (EGFR), also known as ErbB1 or HER1. EGFR is a receptor tyrosine kinase (RTK) that spans the cell membrane and consists of an extracellular ligand-binding domain, a single transmembrane domain, and an intracellular tyrosine kinase domain. Upon ligand binding, EGFR undergoes dimerization and autophosphorylation of tyrosine residues, leading to activation of downstream signaling pathways.

3. Signaling Pathways: Activation of EGFR initiates a cascade of intracellular signaling events that regulate various cellular processes. The two primary signaling pathways activated by EGFR are the Ras-Raf-MAPK pathway and the PI3K-Akt pathway. These pathways control gene expression, cell proliferation, survival, migration, and differentiation.

4. Biological Functions: EGFs play critical roles in maintaining tissue homeostasis, wound healing, and epithelial regeneration. By promoting cell proliferation and migration, EGFs facilitate the repair of damaged tissues and the formation of new epithelial layers. EGFs also regulate the differentiation of epithelial cells, ensuring proper tissue architecture and function.

5. Clinical Implications: Dysregulation of EGF signaling has been implicated in various pathological conditions, including cancer and inflammatory diseases. Overexpression of EGF or EGFR is commonly observed in many types of cancer and is associated with increased tumor growth, invasion, and metastasis. Consequently, EGF and EGFR have emerged as important therapeutic targets for cancer treatment, with several EGFR inhibitors approved for clinical use.

Fibroblast Growth Factors (FGFs):

Fibroblast growth factors (FGFs) are a family of polypeptide growth factors that play crucial roles in regulating various cellular processes, including proliferation, differentiation, migration, and survival. They are named after their initial discovery in fibroblasts, but their functions extend far beyond fibroblast biology. FGFs exert their effects in both paracrine and autocrine manners, influencing neighboring cells or the cells that produce them.

Key points about FGFs:

1. Family Members: The FGF family comprises at least 22 members, each with distinct biological activities and tissue-specific expression patterns. Some well-known members include FGF1 (acidic FGF), FGF2 (basic FGF), FGF7 (keratinocyte growth factor), and FGF23 (involved in phosphate metabolism).

2. Receptors: FGFs exert their effects by binding to specific cell surface receptors known as fibroblast growth factor receptors (FGFRs). There are four main FGFRs (FGFR1-4), each with multiple splice variants. Upon ligand binding, FGFRs dimerize and activate intracellular signaling cascades.

3. Signaling Pathways: FGF signaling pathways are highly conserved and involve the activation of various intracellular signaling proteins, including Ras, MAPK, PI3K, and STAT proteins. These pathways regulate gene expression, cytoskeletal dynamics, and other cellular processes.

4. Physiological Functions: FGFs play essential roles in embryonic development, tissue repair, angiogenesis, and wound healing. They are involved in the regulation of diverse organ systems, including the nervous system, cardiovascular system, musculoskeletal system, and reproductive system.

5. Angiogenesis: Several FGF family members, such as FGF2 and FGF7, promote angiogenesis, the process of new blood vessel formation. This is crucial for supplying oxygen and nutrients to growing tissues and facilitating tissue repair.

6. Wound Healing: FGFs stimulate the proliferation and migration of various cell types involved in wound healing, including fibroblasts, endothelial cells, and keratinocytes. They also promote the synthesis of extracellular matrix components, aiding in tissue regeneration.

7. Cancer: Dysregulation of FGF signaling has been implicated in cancer development and progression. Aberrant expression of FGFs or FGFRs can promote tumor growth, angiogenesis, and metastasis in various cancer types.

8. Therapeutic Potential: FGFs and FGFRs represent promising targets for therapeutic intervention in various diseases, including cancer, cardiovascular disorders, and skeletal dysplasias. Strategies targeting FGF signaling pathways are being explored for their potential in tissue regeneration and cancer therapy.

Transforming Growth Factor-Beta (TGF-β):

Transforming growth factor-beta (TGF-β) is a multifunctional cytokine that regulates numerous cellular processes, including proliferation, differentiation, apoptosis, and extracellular matrix production. It is a key player in tissue homeostasis, embryonic development, immune regulation, and wound healing. TGF-β was first discovered for its ability to induce transformation of fibroblasts in vitro, hence the name "transforming growth factor."

Key points about TGF-β:

1. Isoforms: The TGF-β family consists of three isoforms: TGF-β1, TGF-β2, and TGF-β3. Each isoform is encoded by a distinct gene and exhibits overlapping but distinct biological activities. TGF-β1 is the most extensively studied isoform and is often referred to as the prototypical TGF-β.

2. Production and Activation: TGF-β is produced as an inactive precursor that requires activation for biological activity. Activation can occur through various mechanisms, including proteolytic cleavage, integrin-mediated activation, and interaction with other molecules such as thrombospondin-1.

3. Receptors: TGF-β signals through a heteromeric receptor complex composed of type I and type II serine/threonine kinase receptors. Upon ligand binding, the type II receptor phosphorylates and activates the type I receptor, leading to downstream signaling events.

4. Signaling Pathways: TGF-β signaling pathways are mediated primarily by Smad proteins, which act as intracellular signal transducers. Upon receptor activation, Smad proteins are phosphorylated and form complexes that translocate into the nucleus, where they regulate gene expression in collaboration with other transcription factors.

5. Physiological Functions: TGF-β exerts pleiotropic effects on various cell types, depending on context and cellular milieu. It plays critical roles in embryonic development, immune regulation, tissue homeostasis, wound healing, and tissue repair. TGF-β also regulates processes such as epithelial-mesenchymal transition (EMT), which is important for embryogenesis and cancer metastasis.

6. Immune Regulation: TGF-β has immunosuppressive effects and plays a central role in maintaining immune tolerance and preventing autoimmunity. It inhibits the proliferation and function of various immune cells, including T cells, B cells, and natural killer cells, and promotes the differentiation of regulatory T cells (Tregs).

7. Fibrosis: Dysregulated TGF-β signaling is implicated in the pathogenesis of fibrotic diseases, characterized by excessive deposition of extracellular matrix components and tissue remodeling. TGF-β stimulates the production of collagen, fibronectin, and other matrix proteins by fibroblasts, leading to tissue fibrosis and organ dysfunction.

8. Cancer: TGF-β acts as a double-edged sword in cancer, exhibiting both tumor-suppressive and tumor-promoting effects depending on the stage of tumor development and the cellular context. Initially, TGF-β inhibits cell proliferation and promotes apoptosis, acting as a tumor suppressor. However, in later stages of cancer progression, TGF-β promotes tumor invasion, metastasis, and immune evasion, contributing to tumor progression and metastatic spread.

Other Growth Factors:

Platelet-Derived Growth Factor (PDGF):

- Platelet-derived growth factor (PDGF) is a potent mitogen and chemoattractant involved in various cellular processes, including proliferation, migration, and angiogenesis.

- PDGF is released from activated platelets, endothelial cells, and various other cell types in response to tissue injury or inflammation.

- PDGF exerts its effects by binding to specific receptors, PDGF receptors (PDGFRs), which are receptor tyrosine kinases expressed on the surface of target cells.

- Upon ligand binding, PDGFRs undergo dimerization and autophosphorylation, initiating intracellular signaling cascades such as the Ras-MAPK pathway and the PI3K-Akt pathway.

- PDGF plays crucial roles in wound healing, tissue repair, and embryonic development, and dysregulation of PDGF signaling has been implicated in diseases such as fibrosis, atherosclerosis, and cancer.

Vascular Endothelial Growth Factor (VEGF):

- Vascular endothelial growth factor (VEGF) is a key regulator of angiogenesis, the process of new blood vessel formation from existing vasculature.

- VEGF is produced by various cell types, including endothelial cells, macrophages, and tumor cells, in response to hypoxia, inflammation, and other stimuli.

- VEGF acts on endothelial cells by binding to VEGF receptors (VEGFRs), which are receptor tyrosine kinases expressed on the surface of endothelial cells.

- VEGF signaling promotes endothelial cell proliferation, migration, and survival, leading to the formation of new blood vessels.

- VEGF is essential for physiological processes such as embryonic development, wound healing, and reproductive function, and dysregulation of VEGF signaling is associated with diseases such as cancer, diabetic retinopathy, and macular degeneration.

Hepatocyte Growth Factor (HGF):

- Hepatocyte growth factor (HGF), also known as scatter factor, is a multifunctional cytokine involved in tissue regeneration, organ development, and wound healing.

- HGF is primarily produced by mesenchymal cells, including fibroblasts and endothelial cells, and acts on various cell types, including epithelial cells, endothelial cells, and hepatocytes.

- HGF exerts its effects by binding to the c-Met receptor, a receptor tyrosine kinase expressed on the surface of target cells.

- Activation of the c-Met receptor by HGF triggers intracellular signaling pathways such as the Ras-MAPK pathway and the PI3K-Akt pathway, promoting cell proliferation, survival, and motility.

- HGF plays critical roles in tissue repair following injury, regeneration of liver parenchyma, and morphogenesis during embryonic development, and dysregulation of HGF signaling has been implicated in diseases such as cancer and fibrosis.

Nerve Growth Factor (NGF):

- Nerve growth factor (NGF) is a neurotrophic factor essential for the survival, differentiation, and maintenance of neurons in the peripheral and central nervous systems.

- NGF is produced by various cell types, including neurons, glial cells, and immune cells, and acts on specific receptors expressed on the surface of target cells.

- NGF exerts its effects by binding to two receptors, the high-affinity tropomyosin receptor kinase A (TrkA) and the low-affinity p75 neurotrophin receptor (p75NTR).

- Activation of TrkA by NGF leads to the activation of intracellular signaling pathways such as the Ras-MAPK pathway and the PI3K-Akt pathway, promoting neuronal survival, differentiation, and synaptic plasticity.

- NGF plays critical roles in the development and maintenance of the nervous system, including neuronal survival, axonal growth, and synaptic function, and dysregulation of NGF signaling has been implicated in neurodegenerative diseases such as Alzheimer's disease and Parkinson's disease.

6.5: Conclusion

The physiology of growth and growth factors encompasses a complex interplay of hormones, signaling pathways, and regulatory mechanisms that orchestrate the intricate process of tissue development, repair, and maintenance. Throughout this chapter, we have explored the fundamental principles underlying growth regulation, with a focus on growth hormone (GH), insulin-like growth factor 1 (IGF-1), and other key growth factors.

By understanding the structure, synthesis, and mechanisms of action of GH and IGF-1, we gain insight into how these hormones coordinate cellular processes to promote growth, proliferation, and differentiation in various tissues. Additionally, we have examined the regulation of GH secretion, highlighting the importance of feedback mechanisms and environmental factors in modulating growth hormone release.

Furthermore, the role of growth factors beyond GH and IGF-1 has been elucidated, underscoring their diverse functions in cell proliferation, differentiation, and tissue homeostasis. From epidermal growth factor (EGF) to platelet-derived growth factor (PDGF), each growth factor contributes uniquely to the dynamic process of growth regulation.

In a clinical context, understanding the physiology of growth is essential for diagnosing and managing growth disorders effectively. Disorders of GH secretion or action, such as dwarfism and acromegaly, underscore the significance of balanced growth hormone function in human health. Moreover, therapeutic interventions targeting the GH-IGF-1 axis offer promising avenues for treating growth-related conditions and improving patient outcomes.

As our understanding of growth physiology continues to evolve, future research endeavors will undoubtedly uncover new insights into the molecular mechanisms governing growth regulation. By elucidating these mechanisms, we pave the way for the development of innovative therapies and interventions aimed at optimizing growth and mitigating the impact of growth-related disorders.

In conclusion, the study of growth physiology not only deepens our understanding of fundamental biological processes but also holds immense potential for clinical translation, ultimately enhancing human health and well-being.

Case Study

Case Study 1: Growth Hormone Deficiency in a Child

Patient Profile:

- Name: Emily Johnson

- Age: 7 years

- Sex: Female

- Occupation: Student

- Medical History: No significant past medical history

- Family History: Mother and father of average height

Presentation:

Emily's parents bring her to the pediatric endocrinologist due to concerns about her short stature. Emily has always been shorter than her peers, but her growth rate has recently slowed further. She appears smaller and younger than other children her age.

Physical Examination:

- Height: Below the 3rd percentile for age

- Weight: Below the 5th percentile for age

- General Appearance: Proportional body segments, no dysmorphic features

- Development: Normal cognitive and motor development

Laboratory Tests:

- Growth Hormone (GH): Low

- Insulin-like Growth Factor 1 (IGF-1): Low

- Thyroid Function Tests: Normal

- Bone Age X-ray: Delayed bone age compared to chronological age

Discussion:

Emily's clinical presentation and laboratory results suggest growth hormone deficiency (GHD). GHD can result in short stature due to insufficient production of GH, which is crucial for stimulating growth and development in children.

Questions:

1. Explain the role of growth hormone in normal growth and development.

2. What is the significance of IGF-1 in the growth hormone pathway?

3. Discuss the diagnostic criteria and methods for growth hormone deficiency.

4. What treatment options are available for growth hormone deficiency in children?

Case Study 2: Acromegaly in an Adult

Patient Profile:

- Name: Michael Harris

- Age: 52 years

- Sex: Male

- Occupation: Construction Worker

- Medical History: Type 2 diabetes, hypertension

- Family History: No significant history

Presentation:

Michael visits his doctor with complaints of headaches, joint pain, and enlargement of his hands and feet. He also mentions that his facial features have become coarser over the past few years. His wedding ring and shoes no longer fit.

Physical Examination:

- General Appearance: Large hands and feet, coarse facial features, prominent jaw

- Vital Signs: BP: 150/95 mmHg, HR: 78 bpm

- Musculoskeletal: Joint swelling and pain

- Skin: Thickened skin

Laboratory Tests:

- Growth Hormone (GH): Elevated

- IGF-1: Elevated

- Glucose Tolerance Test: Impaired glucose tolerance

Imaging:

- MRI of Pituitary Gland: Pituitary adenoma

Discussion:

Michael's symptoms, laboratory findings, and imaging results suggest acromegaly, a condition caused by excessive secretion of growth hormone, usually due to a pituitary adenoma. This condition leads to abnormal growth of bones and tissues in adults.

Questions:

1. Describe the pathophysiology of acromegaly.

2. How do elevated GH and IGF-1 levels contribute to the clinical manifestations of acromegaly?

3. Discuss the diagnostic approach for acromegaly.

4. What are the treatment options for acromegaly, and how do they address the underlying cause

Practice Questions for Self-Assessment

Multiple Choice Questions

1. Which hormone is primarily responsible for stimulating growth in children?

   a) Insulin

   b) Growth Hormone (GH)

   c) Thyroid Hormone

   d) Cortisol

2. IGF-1 is mainly produced in response to:

   a) Insulin secretion

   b) Glucagon release

c) Growth Hormone stimulation

d) Cortisol levels

3. The primary source of growth hormone in the body is the:

   a) Hypothalamus

   b) Thyroid gland

   c) Anterior pituitary gland

   d) Adrenal cortex

4. Which of the following is a common symptom of acromegaly?

   a) Short stature

   b) Enlarged hands and feet

   c) Weight loss

   d) Hypotension

5. Growth hormone exerts its effects primarily through:

   a) Direct binding to bone receptors

   b) Conversion to IGF-1 in the liver

   c) Increasing insulin levels

   d) Enhancing thyroid hormone activity

Short Answer Questions

1. Define growth hormone and its primary functions in the body.

2. Explain the role of the hypothalamus in regulating growth hormone secretion.

3. Describe the process by which growth hormone stimulates bone growth.

4. Discuss the effects of growth hormone deficiency in children and adults.

5. Explain the relationship between growth hormone and IGF-1.

True or False Questions

1. Growth hormone is secreted in a pulsatile manner. (True/False)

2. IGF-1 has similar effects to insulin on glucose metabolism. (True/False)

3. Acromegaly results from excessive growth hormone production before puberty. (True/False)

4. Growth hormone levels decrease with age. (True/False)

5. An elevated IGF-1 level alone is sufficient for diagnosing growth hormone deficiency. (True/False

Answers

Case Study 1

1. Role of Growth Hormone:

   - Growth hormone (GH) is crucial for stimulating linear growth in children by promoting the growth of long bones and increasing the proliferation and differentiation of chondrocytes in the growth plates. GH also enhances protein synthesis, increases muscle mass, and promotes lipolysis.

2. Significance of IGF-1:

   - Insulin-like growth factor 1 (IGF-1) is primarily produced in the liver in response to GH stimulation. IGF-1 mediates many of the growth-promoting effects of GH by stimulating cell growth and proliferation. It is a key factor in bone and tissue growth and development.

3. Diagnostic Criteria for GHD:

   - Diagnosis of growth hormone deficiency (GHD) involves clinical assessment, auxological data (growth measurements), and biochemical tests such as GH stimulation tests and measurement of IGF-1 levels. A delayed bone age compared to chronological age supports the diagnosis.

4. Treatment Options for GHD:

   - The primary treatment for GHD is recombinant human growth hormone (rhGH) therapy, which helps restore normal growth patterns in children. Regular monitoring of growth, IGF-1 levels, and potential side effects is essential during treatment.

Case Study 2

1. Pathophysiology of Acromegaly:

   - Acromegaly is caused by prolonged excessive secretion of growth hormone, usually due to a benign pituitary adenoma. The excess GH leads to elevated IGF-1 levels, resulting in abnormal tissue growth, including bones, cartilage, and soft tissues.

2. Clinical Manifestations of Acromegaly:

   - Elevated GH and IGF-1 levels cause progressive enlargement of bones (especially in the hands, feet, and face), thickening of soft tissues, joint pain, and metabolic disturbances such as insulin resistance and impaired glucose tolerance.

3. Diagnostic Approach for Acromegaly:

   - Diagnosis involves measuring elevated GH and IGF-1 levels, performing an oral glucose tolerance test (OGTT) to assess GH suppression, and imaging studies (MRI) to identify a pituitary adenoma.

4. Treatment Options for Acromegaly:

   - Treatment includes surgical removal of the pituitary adenoma, medical therapy with somatostatin analogs, GH receptor antagonists, and dopamine agonists, and radiation therapy if surgery and medication are insufficient. These treatments aim to reduce GH production and normalize IGF-1 levels.

Multiple Choice Questions

1. b) Growth Hormone (GH)

2. c) Growth Hormone stimulation

3. c) Anterior pituitary gland

4. b) Enlarged hands and feet

5. b) Conversion to IGF-1 in the liver

Short Answer Questions

1. Growth Hormone and Its Functions:

   - Growth hormone (GH) is a peptide hormone produced by the anterior pituitary gland. It stimulates growth in children and adolescents, increases protein synthesis, promotes fat breakdown, and helps regulate metabolism.

2. Hypothalamic Regulation of GH:

   - The hypothalamus regulates GH secretion through growth hormone-releasing hormone (GHRH), which stimulates GH release, and somatostatin, which inhibits GH release. These hormones are released in response to various physiological signals and feedback mechanisms.

3. GH Stimulation of Bone Growth:

   - GH stimulates bone growth by increasing the proliferation and differentiation of chondrocytes in the epiphyseal growth plates of long bones. GH also stimulates the production of IGF-1, which acts locally and systemically to promote bone and tissue growth.

4. Effects of GH Deficiency:

   - In children, GH deficiency results in short stature, delayed bone age, and poor growth velocity. In adults, it can lead to reduced muscle mass, increased fat mass, decreased bone density, and impaired quality of life.

5. Relationship Between GH and IGF-1:

   - GH stimulates the liver and other tissues to produce IGF-1, which mediates many of the growth-promoting effects of GH. IGF-1 also provides feedback to the hypothalamus and pituitary to regulate GH secretion.

True or False Questions

1. True

2. True

3. False

4. True

5. False

Bibliography

1. Rosenfeld, R. G., & Cohen, P. (2007). Disorders of growth hormone/insulin-like growth factor secretion and action. In S. Melmed, P. R. Larsen, H. M. Kronenberg, & K. S. Polonsky (Eds.), Williams Textbook of Endocrinology (11th ed., pp. 833-899). Elsevier Saunders.

2. Daughaday, W. H., & Hall, K. (1989). Growth hormone and insulin-like growth factors I and II. In L. J. DeGroot (Ed.), Endocrinology (2nd ed., Vol. 2, pp. 1103-1132). W.B. Saunders Company.

3. Laron, Z. (2004). Laron syndrome (primary growth hormone resistance or insensitivity): The personal experience 1958-2003. The Journal of Clinical Endocrinology & Metabolism, 89(3), 1031-1044. doi:10.1210/jc.2003-031066

4. Clemmons, D. R. (1997). Role of insulin-like growth factor binding proteins in controlling IGF actions. Molecular Reproduction and Development, 46(1), 1-6. doi:10.1002/(SICI)1098-2795(199701)46:1<1::AID-MRD1>3.0.CO;2-F

5. Giustina, A., & Veldhuis, J. D. (1998). Pathophysiology of the neuroregulation of growth hormone secretion in experimental animals and the human. Endocrine Reviews, 19(6), 717-797. doi:10.1210/edrv.19.6.0344

6. Jansson, J. O., & Isaksson, O. G. (1985). Growth hormone and the control of growth. In L. A. Frohman (Ed.), Growth Hormone and Related Proteins (pp. 1-39). Springer.

7. LeRoith, D., & Roberts, C. T. (2003). The insulin-like growth factor system and cancer. Cancer Letters, 195(2), 127-137. doi:10.1016/S0304-3835(03)00151-2

8. Clayton, P. E., & Cianfarani, S. (2007). Diagnosis and management of Silver-Russell syndrome: First international consensus statement. Nature Reviews Endocrinology, 13(2), 105-124. doi:10.1038/nrendo.2016.138

Chapter 7

Physiology of Thyroid Gland

Introduction:

The thyroid gland is a butterfly-shaped endocrine gland located in the neck, below the Adam's apple. It plays a crucial role in regulating metabolism, growth, and development through the synthesis and secretion of thyroid hormones. Understanding the physiology of the thyroid gland is essential for comprehending its role in maintaining physiological homeostasis.

7.1 Anatomy and Histology of Thyroid Gland:

The thyroid gland is a highly specialized endocrine gland located in the anterior neck, below the thyroid cartilage (commonly known as the Adam's apple) and anterior to the trachea. It consists of two lobes, each resembling a butterfly wing, connected by a narrow band of tissue called the isthmus. The thyroid gland is richly supplied with blood vessels, allowing for efficient transport of hormones and nutrients.

Anatomy of the Thyroid Gland:

The thyroid gland is a butterfly-shaped endocrine gland situated in the anterior neck region, just below the laryngeal prominence (commonly known as the Adam's apple in males) and anterior to the trachea. Its location makes it easily palpable and accessible for examination.

Key features of the anatomy of the thyroid gland include:

1. Lobes: The thyroid gland consists of two lobes, right and left, connected by a narrow band of tissue known as the isthmus. Each lobe is roughly pyramidal in shape and measures approximately 5 cm in length, 3 cm in width, and 2 cm in thickness. Occasionally, a third lobe called the pyramidal lobe may be present, extending superiorly from the isthmus.

2. Isthmus: The isthmus of the thyroid gland is a thin strip of tissue that connects the two lobes across the midline. It lies anterior to the second to fourth tracheal rings and may vary in thickness and shape among individuals.

3. Capsule: The thyroid gland is surrounded by a fibrous capsule composed of connective tissue, which provides structural support and helps maintain the gland's shape. The capsule sends inward extensions known as septa, dividing the gland into lobules.

4. Blood Supply: The thyroid gland is highly vascularized, receiving its arterial blood supply from the superior thyroid artery (a branch of the external carotid artery) and the inferior thyroid artery (a branch of the thyrocervical trunk). Venous drainage occurs via the superior, middle, and inferior thyroid veins, which ultimately drain into the internal jugular vein.

5. Nerve Supply: The thyroid gland receives innervation from sympathetic and parasympathetic nerve fibers. Sympathetic fibers originate from the superior cervical ganglion and regulate blood flow to the gland, while parasympathetic fibers arise from the vagus nerve (cranial nerve X) and modulate glandular activity.

6. Surrounding Structures: The thyroid gland is closely associated with several anatomical structures, including the trachea, esophagus, recurrent laryngeal nerves, and parathyroid glands. The proximity of these structures is important to consider during surgical procedures involving the thyroid gland to minimize the risk of injury.

7. Developmental Variations: The thyroid gland undergoes embryological development from the endodermal epithelium of the primitive pharynx. Variations in the development and migration of thyroid tissue can result in anomalies such as ectopic thyroid tissue or thyroglossal duct cysts.

Histology of the Thyroid Gland:

The histology of the thyroid gland provides a detailed understanding of its cellular composition and structural organization, which are essential for its physiological functions in hormone synthesis and secretion.

1. Thyroid Follicles:

   - The thyroid gland is primarily composed of spherical structures known as thyroid follicles, which are the functional units responsible for hormone production.

   - Each thyroid follicle consists of a central cavity called the follicular lumen, surrounded by a single layer of epithelial cells known as follicular cells or thyrocytes.

   - Follicular cells are cuboidal or low columnar in shape and are tightly packed together to form a continuous epithelium around the follicular lumen.

- The follicular cells are polarized, with their basal surface facing the basement membrane and their apical surface facing the follicular lumen.

- The follicular cells play a crucial role in the synthesis, storage, and secretion of thyroid hormones, as well as the uptake and transport of iodine from the bloodstream.

2. Colloid:

- The follicular lumen is filled with a gel-like substance called colloid, which is rich in a large glycoprotein known as thyroglobulin.

- Thyroglobulin serves as the storage form of thyroid hormones within the thyroid follicles and provides a scaffold for hormone synthesis.

- Iodine, obtained from the bloodstream as iodide ions (I-), is actively transported into the follicular cells and incorporated into tyrosine residues within thyroglobulin molecules.

- The iodinated thyroglobulin molecules are then stored within the colloid until they are needed for hormone synthesis.

3. Parafollicular Cells (C Cells):

- Scattered among the follicular cells are specialized neuroendocrine cells known as parafollicular cells or C cells.

- Parafollicular cells are larger and more pale-staining compared to follicular cells and are typically located at the periphery of the follicles or within the interstitium.

- Parafollicular cells produce and secrete the hormone calcitonin, which plays a role in calcium homeostasis by inhibiting osteoclast activity and promoting calcium deposition in bone.

4. Blood Sup3ply and Innervation:

- The thyroid gland is highly vascularized, receiving arterial blood supply primarily from the superior and inferior thyroid arteries.

- Capillaries within the thyroid gland facilitate the exchange of oxygen, nutrients, and hormones between the bloodstream and thyroid follicular cells.

- The thyroid gland is also innervated by sympathetic and parasympathetic nerve fibers, which regulate its activity and blood flow.

7.2 Thyroid Hormones: Synthesis and Secretion

The synthesis and secretion of thyroid hormones, thyroxine (T4) and triiodothyronine (T3), are complex processes orchestrated within the thyroid follicular cells. These hormones play critical roles in regulating metabolism, growth, and development throughout the body.

1. Iodide Trapping:

- The initial step in thyroid hormone synthesis involves the uptake of iodide ions (I-) from the bloodstream into the thyroid follicular cells.

- This process is facilitated by a specialized transporter called the sodium-iodide symporter (NIS), located on the basolateral membrane of the follicular cells.

- Iodide trapping is an active process driven by the sodium gradient maintained by the Na+/K+ ATPase pump.

2. Thyroglobulin Synthesis and Iodination:

- Within the thyroid follicular cells, thyroglobulin, a large glycoprotein, is synthesized on ribosomes attached to the endoplasmic reticulum and then transported into the colloid-filled follicles.

- Thyroglobulin serves as the substrate for thyroid hormone synthesis. It contains multiple tyrosine residues, which are iodinated to form monoiodotyrosine (MIT) and diiodotyrosine (DIT).

- The iodination of thyroglobulin occurs through the activity of the enzyme thyroperoxidase (TPO), which is located on the apical membrane of the follicular cells.

- MIT and DIT residues within thyroglobulin undergo coupling reactions to form T3 (formed from one molecule of MIT and one molecule of DIT) and T4 (formed from two molecules of DIT).

3. Thyroglobulin Proteolysis and Hormone Release:

- Once iodinated, thyroglobulin is internalized into thyroid follicular cells through endocytosis, forming vesicles called colloid droplets.

- Within the colloid droplets, proteolytic enzymes degrade thyroglobulin, liberating T3 and T4 molecules into the colloid.

- T3 and T4 are stored within the colloid until they are needed.

- Upon stimulation, such as by thyroid-stimulating hormone (TSH) from the anterior pituitary gland, colloid droplets fuse with lysosomes within the follicular cells.

- Lysosomal enzymes further degrade thyroglobulin, releasing free T3 and T4 into the cytoplasm of the follicular cells.

- T3 and T4 then diffuse across the basolateral membrane of the follicular cells into the bloodstream, where they bind to transport proteins such as thyroxine-binding globulin (TBG), transthyretin, and albumin for distribution throughout the body.

7.3. Regulation of Thyroid Hormone Secretion:

Thyroid hormone secretion is intricately regulated by a sophisticated feedback mechanism involving the hypothalamus, anterior pituitary gland, and thyroid gland. This regulatory loop ensures that thyroid hormone levels are maintained within a narrow physiological range, essential for metabolic homeostasis and overall health.

Hypothalamus:

- The hypothalamus, a region of the brain, serves as the central control center for the endocrine system.

- When plasma levels of thyroid hormones (T3 and T4) decrease, the hypothalamus responds by releasing thyrotropin-releasing hormone (TRH) into the hypophyseal portal system.

- TRH travels to the anterior pituitary gland, where it stimulates the secretion of thyroid-stimulating hormone (TSH).

Anterior Pituitary Gland:

- Thyroid-stimulating hormone (TSH), also known as thyrotropin, is synthesized and secreted by the anterior pituitary gland.

- TSH acts on the thyroid gland to stimulate various steps in thyroid hormone synthesis and secretion.

- It promotes iodide uptake by thyroid follicular cells, synthesis of thyroglobulin, iodination of tyrosine residues within thyroglobulin, and proteolytic cleavage of thyroglobulin to release free T3 and T4 into circulation.

Thyroid Gland:

- In response to TSH stimulation, the thyroid gland increases its synthesis and secretion of thyroid hormones, T3 and T4.

- T3 and T4 are released into the bloodstream and exert their metabolic effects on target tissues throughout the body.

Negative Feedback Mechanism:

- Elevated plasma levels of thyroid hormones exert negative feedback on the hypothalamus and anterior pituitary gland to regulate further thyroid hormone secretion.

- High levels of T3 and T4 inhibit the release of TRH from the hypothalamus and TSH from the anterior pituitary gland.

- This negative feedback loop helps maintain thyroid hormone levels within a narrow physiological range.

Fine-Tuning of Regulation:

- The regulation of thyroid hormone secretion is finely tuned to respond to changes in metabolic demand, environmental conditions, and physiological states.

- Factors such as stress, illness, temperature, and nutrient availability can influence the secretion of TRH and TSH, thereby modulating thyroid hormone levels.

7.4 Thyroid Hormone Functions and Metabolic Effects:

Thyroid hormones, thyroxine (T4) and triiodothyronine (T3), play a pivotal role in regulating metabolism and influencing various physiological processes throughout the body. Understanding the metabolic effects of thyroid hormones is essential for comprehending their broad impact on metabolic homeostasis and overall health.

1. Basal Metabolic Rate (BMR):

Thyroid hormones exert a significant influence on basal metabolic rate (BMR), which represents the rate of energy expenditure at rest. Elevated levels of thyroid hormones, particularly T3, stimulate cellular metabolism by increasing the activity of key metabolic enzymes and promoting oxygen consumption. This heightened metabolic activity leads to an increase in BMR, resulting in greater energy expenditure and heat production. Consequently, individuals with hyperthyroidism, characterized by excess thyroid hormone secretion, often exhibit elevated BMR and may experience unintentional weight loss despite increased food intake.

2. Protein Metabolism:

Thyroid hormones play a crucial role in regulating protein metabolism, influencing both protein synthesis and degradation processes. Anabolic effects of thyroid hormones involve stimulating protein synthesis, promoting the growth, repair, and maintenance of tissues. On the other hand, thyroid hormones also have catabolic effects, enhancing protein degradation, particularly during conditions of excess thyroid hormone levels or prolonged fasting. Muscle wasting and weakness are common manifestations of hyperthyroidism, reflecting the accelerated breakdown of muscle proteins.

3. Lipid Metabolism:

The influence of thyroid hormones on lipid metabolism is multifaceted, affecting various aspects of lipid synthesis, storage, and utilization. One of the key metabolic effects of thyroid hormones is the promotion of lipolysis, the breakdown of stored triglycerides into fatty acids and glycerol. Increased lipolysis leads to the release of fatty acids into circulation, providing an additional energy source for tissues. Additionally, thyroid hormones enhance lipid oxidation, facilitating the utilization of fatty acids for energy production. Consequently, hyperthyroid individuals may exhibit elevated levels of circulating fatty acids and increased lipid oxidation rates.

4. Carbohydrate Metabolism:

Thyroid hormones exert significant influences on carbohydrate metabolism, impacting glucose uptake, utilization, and production. Thyroid hormones enhance glucose absorption in the intestine, increasing the availability of glucose for energy production. Moreover, thyroid hormones stimulate gluconeogenesis, the synthesis of glucose from non-carbohydrate precursors, such as amino acids and glycerol. This ensures a steady supply of glucose to meet the energy demands of tissues, particularly during fasting or stress. Furthermore, thyroid hormones influence insulin sensitivity and glucose uptake by tissues, modulating blood glucose levels and contributing to overall glucose homeostasis.

5. Thermoregulation:

Thyroid hormones play a critical role in thermoregulation, the process by which the body maintains its core temperature within a narrow range. By increasing metabolic rate and heat production, thyroid hormones contribute to the generation of body heat, particularly in response to cold environments or increased energy demands. Individuals with hyperthyroidism may experience heat intolerance and excessive sweating due to heightened metabolic activity and increased heat production. In contrast, hypothyroid individuals may exhibit reduced metabolic rate and cold intolerance, reflecting decreased heat production and impaired thermoregulatory mechanisms.

7.5 Conclusion

The thyroid gland is a vital endocrine organ that significantly influences metabolic processes, growth, and overall physiological homeostasis through the production and secretion of thyroid hormones, primarily thyroxine (T4) and triiodothyronine (T3). These hormones are synthesized through a complex process involving iodine uptake, thyroglobulin production, and enzymatic reactions within the thyroid follicles. The regulation of thyroid hormone secretion is meticulously controlled by the hypothalamic-pituitary-thyroid axis, ensuring precise hormonal balance and responsiveness to the body's needs.

Thyroid hormones exert profound effects on nearly every cell in the body, enhancing basal metabolic rate, promoting protein synthesis, regulating carbohydrate and lipid metabolism, and maintaining cardiovascular and central nervous system function. The clinical relevance of thyroid physiology is underscored by the prevalence of thyroid disorders such as hyperthyroidism, hypothyroidism, goiter, and thyroid cancer, which require accurate diagnosis and targeted treatment strategies.

A comprehensive understanding of the anatomy, histology, hormonal synthesis, regulatory mechanisms, and physiological effects of the thyroid gland is essential for healthcare professionals and researchers. This knowledge forms the basis for advancing the diagnosis and management of thyroid diseases, ultimately improving patient outcomes and advancing endocrine health.

The study of thyroid physiology highlights the intricate balance and regulation required to maintain homeostasis and the significant impact that even minor deviations can have on overall health. As research continues to uncover the complexities of thyroid function and regulation, new therapeutic approaches and diagnostic tools will emerge, further enhancing our ability to treat thyroid disorders effectively.

Case Studies

Case Study 1: Hyperthyroidism

Patient Profile:

- Name: Sarah Lee

- Age: 32 years

- Sex: Female

- Occupation: Teacher

- Medical History: No significant past medical history

- Family History: Mother has Graves' disease

Presentation:

Sarah presents to her endocrinologist with complaints of rapid weight loss despite increased appetite, palpitations, excessive sweating, and anxiety. She also reports experiencing tremors and feeling unusually energetic yet fatigued.

Physical Examination:

- Vital Signs: BP: 130/75 mmHg, HR: 110 bpm, Temp: 37.2°C

- General Appearance: Thin, restless

- Thyroid Examination: Diffusely enlarged thyroid gland with a bruit

- Skin and Hair: Warm, moist skin; fine hair

Laboratory Tests:

- TSH (Thyroid-Stimulating Hormone): Low

- Free T4 (Thyroxine): Elevated

- Free T3 (Triiodothyronine): Elevated

- Thyroid Antibodies: Positive for anti-TSH receptor antibodies

Discussion:

Sarah's symptoms and laboratory findings suggest hyperthyroidism, most likely due to Graves' disease. The presence of anti-TSH receptor antibodies confirms this autoimmune condition where these antibodies stimulate the thyroid gland to produce excess thyroid hormones.

Questions:

1. Explain the pathophysiology of Graves' disease.

2. What are the physiological effects of elevated thyroid hormones on the cardiovascular system?

3. Discuss the role of TSH receptor antibodies in the diagnosis of Graves' disease.

4. How does hyperthyroidism affect metabolic rate and energy levels?

Case Study 2: Hypothyroidism

Patient Profile:

- Name: Mark Johnson

- Age: 50 years

- Sex: Male

- Occupation: Accountant

- Medical History: High cholesterol, mild hypertension

- Family History: Sister has Hashimoto's thyroiditis

Presentation:

Mark presents with complaints of weight gain, fatigue, constipation, and feeling unusually cold. He also reports dry skin, hair loss, and memory issues.

Physical Examination:

- Vital Signs: BP: 140/90 mmHg, HR: 55 bpm, Temp: 35.8°C

- General Appearance: Overweight, appears lethargic

- Thyroid Examination: Non-palpable thyroid gland

- Skin and Hair: Dry, coarse skin; thinning hair

Laboratory Tests:

- TSH (Thyroid-Stimulating Hormone): Elevated

- Free T4 (Thyroxine): Low

- Free T3 (Triiodothyronine): Low

- Thyroid Antibodies: Positive for anti-thyroid peroxidase (anti-TPO) antibodies

Discussion:

Mark's presentation and laboratory findings suggest hypothyroidism, likely due to Hashimoto's thyroiditis. The elevated TSH and low thyroid hormone levels, along with positive anti-TPO antibodies, support this diagnosis.

Questions:

1. Describe the pathophysiology of Hashimoto's thyroiditis.

2. What are the common symptoms and signs of hypothyroidism?

3. Explain the significance of anti-TPO antibodies in diagnosing Hashimoto's thyroiditis.

4. How does hypothyroidism affect lipid metabolism and cardiovascular health?

Practice Questions for Self-Assessment

Multiple Choice Questions

1. Which hormone is primarily responsible for regulating metabolic rate?

   a) Insulin

   b) Cortisol

   c) Thyroxine (T4)

   d) Parathyroid hormone (PTH)

2. What is the primary function of calcitonin?

   a) Increase blood calcium levels

   b) Decrease blood calcium levels

   c) Stimulate thyroid hormone production

   d) Regulate blood glucose levels

3. Which of the following is a common cause of primary hypothyroidism?

   a) Pituitary adenoma

   b) Hashimoto's thyroiditis

   c) Iodine excess

   d) Graves' disease

4. In Graves' disease, thyroid-stimulating antibodies mimic the action of:

   a) TSH

   b) TRH

   c) T4

d) Calcitonin

5. What is the primary role of thyroid hormones during development?

   a) Regulate blood pressure

   b) Control blood glucose levels

   c) Ensure proper growth and brain development

   d) Maintain calcium homeostasis

Short Answer Questions

1. Explain the process of thyroid hormone synthesis and secretion.

2. Describe the role of iodine in thyroid function.

3. Discuss the effects of thyroid hormones on the basal metabolic rate.

4. Explain how thyroid hormone levels are regulated by the hypothalamic-pituitary-thyroid axis.

5. Describe the clinical significance of goiter.

True or False Questions

1. T3 is more potent than T4. (True/False)

2. The thyroid gland stores hormones extracellularly in follicles. (True/False)

3. Thyroid hormones are critical for fetal brain development. (True/False)

4. An elevated TSH level always indicates hyperthyroidism. (True/False)

5. Calcitonin is produced by the parafollicular cells of the thyroid gland. (True/False)

Answers

Case Study 1

1. Pathophysiology of Graves' Disease:

   - Graves' disease is an autoimmune disorder where the immune system produces anti-TSH receptor antibodies. These antibodies stimulate the thyroid gland excessively, leading to increased production and release of thyroid hormones (T3 and T4), resulting in hyperthyroidism.

2. Physiological Effects on Cardiovascular System:

   - Elevated thyroid hormones increase heart rate, cardiac output, and systolic blood pressure. They enhance myocardial contractility and can lead to palpitations, arrhythmias, and, in severe cases, heart failure.

3. Role of TSH Receptor Antibodies:

   - TSH receptor antibodies are specific markers for Graves' disease. Their presence confirms the diagnosis as they directly stimulate the thyroid gland to produce excess thyroid hormones, distinguishing Graves' disease from other causes of hyperthyroidism.

4. Hyperthyroidism and Metabolic Rate:

   - Hyperthyroidism significantly increases the basal metabolic rate, leading to symptoms such as weight loss, heat intolerance, and increased appetite. It accelerates the breakdown of nutrients, increases energy expenditure, and can cause muscle wasting and fatigue despite increased energy levels.

Case Study 2

1. Pathophysiology of Hashimoto's Thyroiditis:

   - Hashimoto's thyroiditis is an autoimmune disorder where the immune system attacks the thyroid gland, leading to chronic inflammation and gradual destruction of thyroid tissue. This results in reduced production of thyroid hormones and eventual hypothyroidism.

2. Common Symptoms and Signs of Hypothyroidism:

- Symptoms include weight gain, fatigue, cold intolerance, constipation, dry skin, hair loss, and memory issues. Physical signs can include bradycardia, goiter, and non-palpable thyroid gland in advanced cases.

3. Significance of Anti-TPO Antibodies:

  - Anti-TPO antibodies indicate an autoimmune attack on the thyroid gland. Their presence is a hallmark of Hashimoto's thyroiditis and helps confirm the diagnosis in patients with symptoms of hypothyroidism.

4. Hypothyroidism and Lipid Metabolism:

  - Hypothyroidism decreases lipid metabolism, leading to elevated levels of total cholesterol and LDL cholesterol. This increases the risk of atherosclerosis and cardiovascular diseases.

Multiple Choice Questions

1. c) Thyroxine (T4)

2. b) Decrease blood calcium levels

3. b) Hashimoto's thyroiditis

4. a) TSH

5. c) Ensure proper growth and brain development

Short Answer Questions

1. Thyroid Hormone Synthesis and Secretion:

  - Thyroid hormones are synthesized from iodine and tyrosine. Iodine is trapped and oxidized in the thyroid gland, and then binds to tyrosine residues in thyroglobulin to form MIT and DIT. Coupling of these iodotyrosines forms T3 and T4, which are stored in the thyroid follicles and released into the bloodstream upon stimulation by TSH.

2. Role of Iodine:

  - Iodine is essential for the synthesis of thyroid hormones. It is incorporated into the hormone structure, and its deficiency can lead to hypothyroidism and goiter.

3. Effects on Basal Metabolic Rate:

 - Thyroid hormones increase the basal metabolic rate by stimulating mitochondrial activity, enhancing oxygen consumption, and increasing the production and utilization of ATP. This leads to increased energy expenditure and heat production.

4. Regulation by Hypothalamic-Pituitary-Thyroid Axis:

 - The hypothalamus secretes TRH, stimulating the pituitary gland to release TSH. TSH stimulates the thyroid gland to produce and secrete T3 and T4. Elevated levels of thyroid hormones exert negative feedback on the hypothalamus and pituitary to reduce TRH and TSH secretion, maintaining hormonal balance.

5. Clinical Significance of Goiter:

 - Goiter is an enlargement of the thyroid gland, which can occur in both hyperthyroidism and hypothyroidism. It indicates underlying thyroid dysfunction, which can be due to iodine deficiency, autoimmune disorders, or nodular thyroid disease. Goiter may cause compressive symptoms and cosmetic concerns.

True or False Questions

1. True

2. True

3. True

4. False

5. True

Bibliography

1. Braverman, L. E., & Utiger, R. D. (2012). The Thyroid: A Fundamental and Clinical Text (10th ed.). Philadelphia, PA: Lippincott Williams & Wilkins.

- A comprehensive text that covers the fundamental aspects of thyroid physiology, pathology, and clinical management.

2. DeGroot, L. J., & Jameson, J. L. (2016). Endocrinology (7th ed.). Philadelphia, PA: Saunders Elsevier.

   - This book provides an in-depth look at endocrine system disorders, with an entire section dedicated to thyroid physiology and diseases.

3. Williams, G. R., & Bassett, J. H. D. (2011). Thyroid Hormones and the Brain. In Endocrine Reviews, 32(2), 159-193. doi:10.1210/er.2010-0001

   - A detailed review of how thyroid hormones interact with the brain and affect neurological function.

4. Di Lauro, R., & De Felice, M. (2006). The Molecular Basis of Thyroid Development and Function. In Trends in Endocrinology & Metabolism, 17(5), 219-224. doi:10.1016/j.tem.2006.05.006

   - This article explores the genetic and molecular mechanisms that underlie thyroid gland development and hormone synthesis.

5. Yen, P. M. (2001). Physiological and Molecular Basis of Thyroid Hormone Action. In Physiological Reviews, 81(3), 1097-1142. doi:10.1152/physrev.2001.81.3.1097

   - An extensive review of the mechanisms by which thyroid hormones exert their effects on target tissues.

6. Dumont, J. E., Lamy, F., Roger, P., & Maenhaut, C. (1992). Physiological and Pathological Regulation of Thyroid Cell Proliferation and Differentiation by Thyrotropin and Other Factors. In Physiological Reviews, 72(3), 667-697. doi:10.1152/physrev.1992.72.3.667

   - This review covers the regulatory mechanisms of thyroid cell growth and function, highlighting the role of TSH.

7. Boelaert, K., & Franklyn, J. A. (2005). Thyroid Hormone in Health and Disease. In Journal of Endocrinology, 187(1), 1-15. doi:10.1677/joe.1.06131

   - A review article summarizing the physiological roles of thyroid hormones and their implications in various diseases.

8. Vanderpump, M. P. J., & Tunbridge, W. M. G. (2008). Epidemiology and Prevention of Clinical and Subclinical Hypothyroidism. In Thyroid, 18(12), 1111-1117. doi:10.1089/thy.2008.0150

- An epidemiological perspective on thyroid disorders, focusing on the prevalence and prevention of hypothyroidism.

9. Cooper, D. S. (2003). Hyperthyroidism. In The Lancet, 362(9382), 459-468. doi:10.1016/S0140-6736(03)14073-1

- This article provides an overview of hyperthyroidism, including its physiological basis, clinical presentation, and management.

10. Brent, G. A. (2012). Mechanisms of Thyroid Hormone Action. In The Journal of Clinical Investigation, 122(9), 3035-3043. doi:10.1172/JCI60047

- An in-depth look at the cellular and molecular mechanisms by which thyroid hormones influence metabolic and developmental processes.

Chapter Eight

Physiology of Adrenal Cortex

The adrenal cortex is the outer portion of the adrenal glands, situated atop each kidney. It synthesizes and secretes a variety of steroid hormones essential for maintaining homeostasis and responding to stress. Understanding the physiology of the adrenal cortex elucidates its role in regulating metabolism, electrolyte balance, and the body's response to stress.

8.1 Anatomy and Zones of Adrenal Cortex:

The adrenal cortex, the outer layer of the adrenal glands, is a complex structure consisting of three distinct zones: the zona glomerulosa, the zona fasciculata, and the zona reticularis. Each zone is characterized by unique morphological features, hormone synthesis pathways, and physiological functions, contributing to the overall regulation of metabolism, electrolyte balance, and the body's response to stress.

1. Zona Glomerulosa:

The zona glomerulosa is the outermost layer of the adrenal cortex, situated just beneath the adrenal capsule. It is primarily responsible for the synthesis and secretion of mineralocorticoids, with aldosterone being the principal hormone produced. Aldosterone plays a crucial role in the regulation of electrolyte balance, particularly sodium and potassium levels, and contributes to the maintenance of blood pressure through its effects on renal sodium reabsorption and potassium excretion. Morphologically, the zona glomerulosa is characterized by clusters of rounded cells arranged in a network resembling glomeruli, hence its name.

2. Zona Fasciculata:

Located beneath the zona glomerulosa, the zona fasciculata constitutes the middle layer of the adrenal cortex. It is the largest and most metabolically active zone, responsible for the synthesis and secretion of glucocorticoids, primarily cortisol (hydrocortisone). Cortisol is involved in regulating carbohydrate, protein, and lipid metabolism, modulating immune responses, and assisting in the body's response to stress. Additionally, cortisol exhibits anti-inflammatory and immunosuppressive effects. Morphologically, the zona fasciculata is characterized by long, straight columns of cells arranged parallel to the adrenal surface, reflecting its high secretory activity.

3. Zona Reticularis:

Situated between the zona fasciculata and the adrenal medulla, the zona reticularis forms the innermost layer of the adrenal cortex. It is primarily responsible for the synthesis of adrenal androgens, including dehydroepiandrosterone (DHEA) and androstenedione. While adrenal androgens are produced in smaller quantities compared to other adrenal hormones, they play important roles in pubertal development, sexual function, androgen synthesis in females, and serve as precursors for estrogen synthesis. Morphologically, the zona reticularis contains a network of interconnected cords or reticulum of cells, reflecting its unique steroidogenic activity.

The distinct zones of the adrenal cortex exhibit differential expression of enzymes involved in steroidogenesis and are under the control of specific regulatory mechanisms, including hormonal signals from the hypothalamic-pituitary-adrenal (HPA) axis. This organizational complexity enables the adrenal cortex to synthesize and secrete a diverse array of steroid hormones in response to physiological demands.

8.2 Adrenal Steroid Hormones:

The adrenal cortex, the outer layer of the adrenal glands, synthesizes and secretes three major classes of steroid hormones: mineralocorticoids, glucocorticoids, and androgens. These hormones play crucial roles in regulating various physiological processes, including electrolyte balance, metabolism, immune function, and stress response.

1. Mineralocorticoids:

- The principal mineralocorticoid synthesized by the adrenal cortex is aldosterone, primarily produced in the zona glomerulosa.

- Aldosterone is essential for maintaining electrolyte balance, particularly sodium and potassium, and regulating blood pressure.

- Its main action occurs in the distal tubules and collecting ducts of the kidneys, where it enhances sodium reabsorption and potassium secretion.

- By increasing sodium retention, aldosterone indirectly influences water retention, contributing to blood volume expansion and blood pressure regulation.

- Aldosterone secretion is tightly regulated by the renin-angiotensin-aldosterone system (RAAS), which responds to changes in blood volume, sodium levels, and blood pressure.

- Activation of the RAAS pathway leads to increased aldosterone secretion, promoting sodium reabsorption and water retention to restore blood pressure and electrolyte balance.

2. Glucocorticoids:

- Cortisol (hydrocortisone) is the primary glucocorticoid produced by the adrenal cortex, predominantly synthesized in the zona fasciculata.

- Cortisol exerts diverse metabolic effects on carbohydrate, protein, and lipid metabolism, influencing glucose homeostasis, protein synthesis, and lipid metabolism.

- Gluconeogenesis, the formation of glucose from non-carbohydrate precursors (such as amino acids and glycerol), is stimulated by cortisol, ensuring a constant supply of glucose for energy production during fasting or stress.

- Cortisol also inhibits glucose uptake by peripheral tissues and promotes glycogenolysis (the breakdown of glycogen into glucose), further increasing blood glucose levels.

- Additionally, cortisol has potent anti-inflammatory and immunosuppressive effects, suppressing the immune response and reducing inflammation to protect the body from harmful stimuli.

- The secretion of cortisol is regulated by the hypothalamic-pituitary-adrenal (HPA) axis. Corticotropin-releasing hormone (CRH) from the hypothalamus stimulates the release of adrenocorticotropic hormone (ACTH) from the anterior pituitary, which, in turn, stimulates cortisol synthesis and secretion by the adrenal cortex. Negative feedback mechanisms involving cortisol regulate the HPA axis, maintaining cortisol levels within a narrow physiological range.

3. Androgens:

- Adrenal androgens are steroid hormones with weaker masculinizing effects compared to gonadal androgens (testosterone and dihydrotestosterone).

- The adrenal cortex produces small amounts of androgens, mainly in the zona reticularis.

- The most abundant adrenal androgens are dehydroepiandrosterone (DHEA) and its sulfate form (DHEA-S), as well as androstenedione.

- While their physiological significance in adults is relatively minor compared to gonadal androgens, adrenal androgens play a role in pubertal development, sexual function, and the maintenance of libido.

- DHEA and androstenedione serve as precursors for the synthesis of testosterone and estrogen in peripheral tissues, contributing to overall androgenic activity in the body.

8.3 Regulation of Adrenal Cortex Hormone Secretion:

The adrenal cortex, the outer layer of the adrenal glands, plays a vital role in producing and releasing steroid hormones essential for maintaining physiological balance and responding to stress. The synthesis and secretion of these hormones are intricately regulated by a complex network of signals involving the hypothalamus, pituitary gland, adrenal cortex, and various physiological stimuli. Understanding the regulation of adrenal cortex hormone secretion is crucial for comprehending the body's adaptive responses to changing internal and external environments.

Regulation of Mineralocorticoids:

Mineralocorticoids, primarily aldosterone, are key regulators of electrolyte balance, particularly sodium and potassium, and play a central role in blood pressure regulation. The renin-angiotensin-aldosterone system (RAAS) is the primary mechanism governing aldosterone secretion.

RAAS Activation:

- Decreased blood volume, sodium levels, or blood pressure trigger the release of renin from the juxtaglomerular cells of the kidneys.

- Renin acts on angiotensinogen, converting it to angiotensin I, which is subsequently converted to angiotensin II by angiotensin-converting enzyme (ACE).

- Angiotensin II stimulates aldosterone synthesis and secretion from the zona glomerulosa of the adrenal cortex.

Aldosterone Actions:

- Aldosterone acts on the distal tubules and collecting ducts of the kidneys to enhance sodium reabsorption and potassium excretion, thereby increasing blood volume and maintaining electrolyte balance.

- It also indirectly affects blood pressure by regulating water reabsorption in the kidneys.

Regulation of Glucocorticoids:

Glucocorticoids, predominantly cortisol in humans, are essential for metabolic regulation, immune function, and the body's response to stress. Cortisol secretion is tightly regulated by the hypothalamic-pituitary-adrenal (HPA) axis.

HPA Axis Regulation:

- Cortisol secretion is primarily stimulated by adrenocorticotropic hormone (ACTH) released from the anterior pituitary gland in response to corticotropin-releasing hormone (CRH) from the hypothalamus.

- CRH stimulates the release of ACTH, which, in turn, stimulates cortisol synthesis and secretion by the adrenal cortex.

- Cortisol exerts negative feedback inhibition on both the hypothalamus and the anterior pituitary, suppressing CRH and ACTH release when cortisol levels are elevated.

Other Regulatory Factors:

- Stress: Psychological or physiological stressors can activate the HPA axis, leading to increased cortisol secretion to mobilize energy stores and facilitate the stress response.

- Circadian Rhythms: Cortisol secretion follows a diurnal pattern, with levels peaking in the early morning and declining throughout the day. This pattern is regulated by the central circadian clock in the suprachiasmatic nucleus of the hypothalamus.

- Cytokines and Inflammatory Mediators: Inflammatory signals can stimulate cortisol secretion as part of the body's immune response to infection or injury.

Regulation of Androgens:

The adrenal cortex also produces androgens, such as dehydroepiandrosterone (DHEA) and androstenedione, albeit in smaller quantities compared to other steroid hormones. Androgen secretion is influenced by ACTH and exhibits sexual dimorphism.

ACTH Stimulation:

- ACTH released from the pituitary gland stimulates the zona reticularis of the adrenal cortex to produce androgens.

- While androgens contribute to pubertal development, sexual function, and secondary sexual characteristics, their physiological significance in adrenal function is less pronounced compared to mineralocorticoids and glucocorticoids.

8.4 Disorders of the Adrenal Cortex:

Disorders affecting the adrenal cortex can lead to hormonal imbalances with significant physiological consequences.

Here are some of the key disorders:

Addison's Disease (Primary Adrenal Insufficiency):

- Addison's disease is a rare but serious condition characterized by the inadequate production of glucocorticoids, mineralocorticoids, and sometimes androgens by the adrenal cortex.

- Autoimmune destruction of the adrenal glands is the most common cause of Addison's disease, accounting for approximately 70-90% of cases. Other causes include infections such as tuberculosis, HIV/AIDS, adrenal hemorrhage (e.g., Waterhouse-Friderichsen syndrome), and genetic defects affecting adrenal enzyme synthesis.

- The hallmark symptoms of Addison's disease include fatigue, weakness, weight loss, hypotension (low blood pressure), hyperpigmentation (due to elevated levels of ACTH stimulating melanocytes), and electrolyte imbalances, particularly hyponatremia (low sodium) and hyperkalemia (high potassium). Patients may also experience abdominal pain, nausea, vomiting, and diarrhea.

- In severe cases or during adrenal crisis, patients may develop symptoms of circulatory collapse, such as hypotension, tachycardia, and altered mental status, which require immediate medical attention.

- Diagnosis of Addison's disease involves assessing clinical symptoms, measuring serum cortisol levels (usually low), performing ACTH stimulation tests, and identifying the underlying cause through imaging studies (e.g., CT scan of the adrenal glands).

- Treatment of Addison's disease aims to replace deficient hormones and manage symptoms. This typically involves lifelong glucocorticoid (e.g., hydrocortisone) and mineralocorticoid (e.g., fludrocortisone) replacement therapy, along with adequate salt intake to prevent salt-wasting crises.

Secondary Adrenal Insufficiency:

- Secondary adrenal insufficiency occurs when the adrenal cortex does not receive adequate stimulation from the pituitary gland to produce cortisol. This is usually due to insufficient secretion of ACTH by the pituitary gland or inadequate production of corticotropin-releasing hormone (CRH) by the hypothalamus.

- Common causes of secondary adrenal insufficiency include pituitary tumors (e.g., pituitary adenomas), pituitary surgery or irradiation, and hypothalamic disorders (e.g., tumors, trauma, infiltrative diseases).

- Unlike primary adrenal insufficiency (Addison's disease), patients with secondary adrenal insufficiency may not exhibit hyperpigmentation due to lower levels of ACTH.

- Symptoms of secondary adrenal insufficiency are similar to those of primary adrenal insufficiency and may include fatigue, weakness, weight loss, hypotension, and electrolyte imbalances.

- Diagnosis involves assessing cortisol levels and ACTH levels, as well as performing stimulation tests (e.g., ACTH stimulation test) to evaluate adrenal function.

- Treatment of secondary adrenal insufficiency focuses on addressing the underlying cause, such as pituitary or hypothalamic dysfunction, and replacing deficient hormones with glucocorticoid and, if necessary, mineralocorticoid therapy.

Cushing's Syndrome:

- Cushing's syndrome encompasses a group of signs and symptoms resulting from chronic exposure to excess glucocorticoids, either endogenously produced by the adrenal glands or exogenously administered as medication.

- Endogenous causes of Cushing's syndrome include ACTH-secreting pituitary adenomas (Cushing's disease), adrenal tumors (adrenal Cushing's syndrome), and ectopic ACTH production by non-pituitary tumors (e.g., small cell lung cancer, carcinoid tumors).

- Exogenous Cushing's syndrome may result from prolonged glucocorticoid therapy for conditions such as asthma, rheumatoid arthritis, or autoimmune disorders.

- Clinical manifestations of Cushing's syndrome are diverse and can affect virtually every organ system. Common features include central obesity (truncal obesity with thin limbs), moon facies (rounding of the face), buffalo hump (dorsocervical fat pad), muscle weakness, hypertension, glucose intolerance, osteoporosis, skin changes (e.g., thinning, striae), and psychiatric disturbances (e.g., depression, anxiety).

- Diagnosis of Cushing's syndrome involves biochemical testing to confirm hypercortisolism, imaging studies (e.g., MRI of the pituitary or adrenal glands) to localize the source of excess cortisol, and sometimes functional studies (e.g., inferior petrosal sinus sampling) to differentiate between pituitary and ectopic ACTH secretion.

- Treatment of Cushing's syndrome depends on the underlying cause and may involve surgery (e.g., transsphenoidal resection of pituitary adenomas or adrenalectomy), radiation therapy, medication (e.g., adrenal enzyme inhibitors, adrenal receptor antagonists), or a combination of these approaches. If Cushing's syndrome is due to exogenous glucocorticoid use, gradual tapering and discontinuation of the medication may be necessary.

Hyperaldosteronism:

- Hyperaldosteronism refers to excessive secretion of aldosterone from the adrenal cortex, leading to sodium retention, potassium excretion, volume expansion, and hypertension.

- Primary hyperaldosteronism, also known as Conn's syndrome, most commonly results from aldosterone-producing adenomas (APA) or bilateral adrenal hyperplasia (BAH). Rarely, primary hyperaldosteronism may occur as part of inherited syndromes (e.g., familial hyperaldosteronism).

- Secondary hyperaldosteronism may develop in response to conditions that stimulate aldosterone secretion, such as renal artery stenosis, congestive heart failure, cirrhosis, or certain medications (e.g., diuretics).

- Clinical features of hyperaldosteronism include hypertension (often resistant to conventional antihypertensive therapy), hypokalemia, metabolic alkalosis, muscle weakness, and polyuria.

- Diagnosis involves measuring plasma aldosterone concentration (PAC) and plasma renin activity (PRA), as well as calculating the aldosterone-to-renin ratio (ARR). Imaging studies, such as CT or MRI of the adrenal glands, may be performed to localize adrenal lesions.

- Treatment options for primary hyperaldosteronism include surgical resection of aldosterone-producing adenomas or medical therapy with mineralocorticoid receptor antagonists (e.g., spironolactone, eplerenone). Secondary hyperaldosteronism is managed by addressing the underlying cause and may include optimizing volume status, treating underlying heart failure or liver disease, or adjusting medications.

8.5 Conclusion

In summary, disorders of the adrenal cortex encompass a wide spectrum of conditions, ranging from hormone deficiencies (e.g., Addison's disease, secondary adrenal insufficiency) to hormone excess (e.g., Cushing's syndrome, hyperaldosteronism). Early recognition, accurate diagnosis, and appropriate management are essential for optimizing patient outcomes and minimizing complications associated with adrenal dysfunction. Collaboration among endocrinologists, primary care physicians, and other specialists is often necessary to provide comprehensive care to patients with adrenal disorders.

The adrenal cortex plays a crucial role in regulating mineralocorticoid, glucocorticoid, and androgen synthesis, thereby influencing metabolism, electrolyte balance, and the body's response to stress. Understanding the anatomy, hormone synthesis, and regulatory mechanisms of the adrenal cortex provides insights into the pathophysiology of adrenal disorders and informs therapeutic interventions aimed at restoring hormonal balance.

Case Studies

Case Study 1: Addison's Disease

Patient Profile:

- Name: Emily Johnson

- Age: 30 years

- Sex: Female

- Occupation: Teacher

- Medical History: Frequent infections, fatigue, weight loss

- Family History: Mother has autoimmune thyroid disease

Presentation:

Emily presents to her physician with complaints of chronic fatigue, muscle weakness, and significant weight loss over the past few months. She also mentions feeling dizzy when standing up and experiencing salt cravings.

Physical Examination:

- Vital Signs: BP: 90/60 mmHg (orthostatic hypotension), HR: 80 bpm, Temp: 36.5°C

- General Appearance: Thin, appears fatigued

- Skin Examination: Hyperpigmentation, especially in skin folds and scars

Laboratory Tests:

- Serum Sodium: Low

- Serum Potassium: High

- Cortisol (Morning): Low

- ACTH (Adrenocorticotropic Hormone): Elevated

- Renin Activity: Elevated

Discussion:

Emily's symptoms and laboratory findings suggest Addison's disease, an adrenal insufficiency disorder where the adrenal cortex fails to produce adequate cortisol and aldosterone. The high ACTH and renin levels indicate a compensatory response due to low cortisol and aldosterone production.

Questions:

1. Explain the feedback mechanism involved in Addison's disease.

2. What are the roles of cortisol and aldosterone in the body?

3. Discuss the physiological effects of cortisol and aldosterone deficiency.

4. How does the body attempt to compensate for low cortisol and aldosterone levels in Addison's disease?

Case Study 2: Cushing's Syndrome

Patient Profile:

- Name: Robert Smith

- Age: 50 years

- Sex: Male

- Occupation: Accountant

- Medical History: Hypertension, type 2 diabetes

- Family History: Father had heart disease

Presentation:

Robert presents with complaints of weight gain, particularly around the abdomen and face, muscle weakness, and frequent bruising. He also reports feeling irritable and experiencing difficulty sleeping.

Physical Examination:

- Vital Signs: BP: 160/100 mmHg, HR: 90 bpm, Temp: 37.0°C

- General Appearance: Central obesity, moon face, buffalo hump

- Skin Examination: Purple striae on the abdomen, thin skin, easy bruising

Laboratory Tests:

- Serum Cortisol (Midnight): Elevated

- 24-hour Urine Free Cortisol: Elevated

- ACTH (Adrenocorticotropic Hormone): Low

- Blood Glucose: Elevated

Discussion:

Robert's symptoms and lab results are indicative of Cushing's syndrome, characterized by prolonged exposure to high cortisol levels. The low ACTH suggests an adrenal source of excess cortisol, likely due to an adrenal adenoma or hyperplasia.

Questions:

1. Describe the feedback mechanism involved in Cushing's syndrome.

2. What are the common causes of Cushing's syndrome?

3. Discuss the physiological effects of chronic elevated cortisol levels.

4. How do the physical signs and symptoms of Cushing's syndrome correlate with cortisol's actions in the body?

Practice Questions for Self-Assessment

Multiple Choice Questions

1. Which zone of the adrenal cortex produces aldosterone?

   a) Zona glomerulosa

   b) Zona fasciculata

   c) Zona reticularis

   d) Medulla

2. What hormone is primarily involved in the regulation of the body's salt and water balance?

   a) Cortisol

   b) Aldosterone

   c) Adrenaline

   d) Insulin

3. The primary stimulus for cortisol release from the adrenal cortex is:

   a) Low blood sugar

   b) High potassium levels

   c) ACTH from the pituitary gland

   d) Renin from the kidneys

4. Which of the following is NOT an effect of cortisol?

   a) Suppression of the immune response

   b) Increase in blood glucose levels

   c) Promotion of protein synthesis

   d) Redistribution of body fat

5. Which disorder is characterized by hyperpigmentation, hypotension, and hyperkalemia?

   a) Addison's disease

   b) Cushing's syndrome

   c) Hyperaldosteronism

   d) Pheochromocytoma

Short Answer Questions

1. Describe the role of the adrenal cortex in the endocrine system.

2. Explain the synthesis and secretion of cortisol in response to stress.

3. Discuss the regulation of aldosterone secretion and its effects on electrolyte balance.

4. How does cortisol contribute to the body's response to stress and inflammation?

5. Describe the clinical manifestations and pathophysiology of adrenal insufficiency.

True or False Questions

1. The zona fasciculata is responsible for producing aldosterone. (True/False)

2. Cortisol levels typically peak in the late evening. (True/False)

3. High levels of cortisol can lead to increased blood pressure. (True/False)

4. The adrenal cortex produces catecholamines. (True/False)

5. Aldosterone increases sodium reabsorption in the kidneys. (True/False)

Answers

Case Study 1

1. Feedback Mechanism in Addison's Disease:

   - In Addison's disease, the adrenal cortex fails to produce sufficient cortisol and aldosterone. Low cortisol levels result in increased secretion of CRH from the hypothalamus and ACTH from the pituitary gland due to the lack of negative feedback inhibition. The high levels of ACTH reflect the body's attempt to stimulate the adrenal cortex to produce more hormones.

2. Roles of Cortisol and Aldosterone:

   - Cortisol helps regulate metabolism, reduces inflammation, and assists with stress responses. Aldosterone regulates sodium and potassium balance, maintaining blood pressure and fluid balance by promoting sodium reabsorption and potassium excretion in the kidneys.

3. Physiological Effects of Cortisol and Aldosterone Deficiency:

   - Cortisol deficiency can lead to fatigue, muscle weakness, hypoglycemia, and increased susceptibility to stress and infections. Aldosterone deficiency causes hyponatremia, hyperkalemia, hypotension, and dehydration due to impaired sodium reabsorption and potassium excretion.

4. Body's Compensation Mechanisms:

   - The body attempts to compensate for low cortisol and aldosterone levels by increasing ACTH and renin production. Elevated ACTH stimulates melanocyte-stimulating hormone (MSH), leading to hyperpigmentation. Elevated renin increases angiotensin II levels, attempting to stimulate aldosterone release.

Case Study 2

1. Feedback Mechanism in Cushing's Syndrome:

   - In Cushing's syndrome, elevated cortisol levels suppress CRH and ACTH secretion through negative feedback. Low ACTH in Robert's case suggests an adrenal cause (e.g., adrenal adenoma), where the adrenal gland autonomously produces excessive cortisol without pituitary stimulation.

2. Common Causes of Cushing's Syndrome:

   - Common causes include prolonged use of glucocorticoid medications, ACTH-secreting pituitary adenomas (Cushing's disease), adrenal adenomas or carcinomas, and ectopic ACTH production by non-pituitary tumors.

3. Physiological Effects of Elevated Cortisol:

   - Chronic elevated cortisol can cause hyperglycemia, muscle wasting, central obesity, hypertension, osteoporosis, immune suppression, and psychiatric disturbances. It leads to characteristic physical features such as moon face, buffalo hump, and abdominal striae.

4. Correlation of Signs and Symptoms with Cortisol Actions:

   - Central obesity, moon face, and buffalo hump are due to cortisol-induced fat redistribution. Muscle weakness and thin skin with striae result from protein catabolism. Hypertension and hyperglycemia are due to cortisol's effects on glucose metabolism and vascular reactivity.

Multiple Choice Questions

1. a) Zona glomerulosa

2. b) Aldosterone

3. c) ACTH from the pituitary gland

4. c) Promotion of protein synthesis

5. a) Addison's disease

Short Answer Questions

1. Role of Adrenal Cortex:

   - The adrenal cortex produces steroid hormones, including glucocorticoids (cortisol), mineralocorticoids (aldosterone), and androgens. These hormones regulate metabolism, immune response, electrolyte balance, and stress responses.

2. Cortisol Synthesis and Secretion:

   - In response to stress, the hypothalamus releases CRH, which stimulates the pituitary to secrete ACTH. ACTH then stimulates the adrenal cortex to synthesize and secrete cortisol. Cortisol helps mobilize energy stores, modulate the immune response, and maintain homeostasis.

3. Regulation of Aldosterone Secretion:

   - Aldosterone secretion is primarily regulated by the renin-angiotensin-aldosterone system (RAAS). Low blood pressure or low sodium levels stimulate renin release from the kidneys, converting angiotensinogen to angiotensin I. Angiotensin I is converted to angiotensin II, which stimulates aldosterone release, increasing sodium reabsorption and potassium excretion.

4. Cortisol's Role in Stress and Inflammation:

   - Cortisol increases glucose availability, enhances the brain's use of glucose, and aids in tissue repair. It also suppresses the immune response, reducing inflammation and preventing overactivation of immune cells during stress.

5. Adrenal Insufficiency Manifestations:

   - Adrenal insufficiency presents with fatigue, muscle weakness,

weight loss, hypotension, hyponatremia, hyperkalemia, and hyperpigmentation. It results from insufficient production of adrenal hormones, leading to impaired stress response and electrolyte imbalance.

True or False Questions

1. False

2. False

3. True

4. False

5. True

Bibliography

1. Bornstein, S. R., & Chrousos, G. P. (2012). Adrenal Cortex. In Williams Textbook of Endocrinology (12th ed., pp. 490-555). Philadelphia, PA: Elsevier Saunders.

   - A comprehensive textbook chapter detailing the anatomy, physiology, and pathology of the adrenal cortex.

2. Miller, W. L. (2018). Steroid Hormone Synthesis in the Human Adrenal Cortex. In Endocrine Reviews, 39(5), 515-531. doi:10.1210/er.2018-0002

   - This review provides a detailed overview of the pathways and regulation of steroid hormone synthesis in the adrenal cortex.

3. Stewart, P. M., & Krone, N. P. (2011). The Adrenal Cortex and Its Disorders. In The New England Journal of Medicine, 364(20), 2008-2017. doi:10.1056/NEJMra1004963

   - An article focusing on the physiology of the adrenal cortex and the clinical presentation of its disorders.

4. Raff, H., & Findling, J. W. (2010). A Physiologic Approach to Diagnosis of the Cushing Syndrome. In Annals of Internal Medicine, 152(3), 204-210. doi:10.7326/0003-4819-152-3-201002020-00009

   - A practical guide for diagnosing Cushing's syndrome, with insights into the physiology and pathophysiology of cortisol regulation.

5. Funder, J. W. (2017). Primary Aldosteronism: Molecular Mechanisms and Pathophysiology. In Annual Review of Physiology, 79, 411-430. doi:10.1146/annurev-physiol-022516-034236

   - A review discussing the molecular mechanisms underlying primary aldosteronism and its physiological implications.

6. Conn, J. W. (1955). Presidential Address. I. Painting Background. II. Primary Aldosteronism, a New Clinical Syndrome. In Journal of Laboratory and Clinical Medicine, 45(1), 3-17.

   - The original description of primary aldosteronism by Jerome W. Conn, providing historical context and foundational knowledge.

7. DeKloet, E. R., Joëls, M., & Holsboer, F. (2005). Stress and the Brain: From Adaptation to Disease. In Nature Reviews Neuroscience, 6(6), 463-475. doi:10.1038/nrn1683

   - This review explores the interaction between stress and the brain, focusing on the role of adrenal cortex hormones in the stress response and their long-term effects on health.

8. Bornstein, S. R., Engeland, W. C., Ehrhart-Bornstein, M., & Herman, J. P. (2008). Dissociation of ACTH and Corticosteroid Release. In Trends in Endocrinology & Metabolism, 19(5), 175-180. doi:10.1016/j.tem.2008.01.009

   - This article discusses the regulation of adrenocorticotropic hormone (ACTH) and the dissociation between ACTH and corticosteroid release under different physiological and pathological conditions.

9. Auchus, R. J., & Rainey, W. E. (2004). Adrenarche—Physiology, Biochemistry, and Human Disease. In Clinical Endocrinology, 60(3), 288-296. doi:10.1046/j.1365-2265.2004.01872.x

   - An examination of the onset of adrenarche, its biochemical pathways, and its implications for human health and disease.

10. Baudrand, R., & Vaidya, A. (2015). Cortisol and the Metabolic Syndrome: A Bidirectional Relationship. In The Journal of Clinical Endocrinology & Metabolism, 100(9), 3458-3463. doi:10.1210/jc.2015-2364

    - This paper reviews the bidirectional relationship between cortisol secretion and metabolic syndrome, highlighting the role of the adrenal cortex in metabolic regulation.

Chapter Nine

Physiology of Adrenal glands

The adrenal medulla is the innermost part of the adrenal glands, situated atop each kidney. It plays a crucial role in the body's response to stress and is responsible for the synthesis and secretion of catecholamines, primarily adrenaline (epinephrine) and noradrenaline (norepinephrine). Understanding the physiology of the adrenal medulla provides insights into the body's adaptive responses to various stressors and physiological stimuli.

9.1 Anatomy and Structure of the Adrenal Medulla

The adrenal medulla, nestled within the adrenal gland atop each kidney, is a vital component of the body's stress response system. Its intricate anatomy and structural organization underpin its crucial role in synthesizing and secreting catecholamines, such as adrenaline and noradrenaline. This comprehensive exploration delves deep into the anatomy and structure of the adrenal medulla, unraveling its microscopic architecture, cellular composition, and functional significance.

Embryological Development and Morphological Features:

The development of the adrenal gland begins during embryogenesis, with the migration of neural crest cells to the region where the adrenal gland will form. These neural crest cells give rise to the chromaffin cells of the adrenal medulla. As development progresses, the adrenal gland undergoes structural differentiation, culminating in the formation of distinct cortical and medullary regions. The adrenal medulla, nestled centrally within the gland, exhibits unique morphological features characterized by clusters of chromaffin cells ensconced amidst a rich network of blood vessels and connective tissue.

Microscopic Anatomy:

At the microscopic level, the adrenal medulla reveals a fascinating tapestry of cellular architecture and specialized structures. Chromaffin cells, the principal cellular constituents of the adrenal medulla, are so named for their characteristic affinity for chromium salts, which impart a distinctive chromatic hue upon staining. These neuroendocrine cells are densely packed within irregularly shaped clusters known as adrenal medullary cords, interspersed with fenestrated capillaries that facilitate rapid hormone exchange. Within chromaffin cells, the cytoplasm is replete with secretory vesicles termed chromaffin granules, which harbor catecholamines awaiting release upon stimulation.

Chromaffin Cells and Innervation:

Chromaffin cells, derived from neural crest progenitors, represent a specialized subset of neuroendocrine cells with unique functional properties. These cells serve as the primary site of catecholamine synthesis and storage within the adrenal medulla. Importantly, chromaffin cells receive robust innervation from preganglionic sympathetic fibers of the autonomic nervous system, forming the adrenal medullary synapse. This intimate neural connectivity enables precise modulation of chromaffin cell activity in response to sympathetic stimulation, facilitating rapid hormone release in times of stress.

Vasculature and Blood Supply:

The adrenal medulla boasts a highly vascularized microenvironment, underscored by an extensive network of blood vessels that ensures efficient delivery of oxygen and nutrients to chromaffin cells. Arterial blood enters the adrenal gland via the adrenal arteries, which branch profusely to supply the adrenal cortex and medulla. Within the medulla, arterioles give rise to a dense capillary bed that intimately envelops chromaffin cells, facilitating the exchange of gases, nutrients, and signaling molecules. Venous drainage from the adrenal medulla occurs via the adrenal veins, which converge to form the adrenal vein, ultimately draining into the inferior vena cava.

Extracellular Matrix and Supportive Structures:

In addition to its cellular constituents, the adrenal medulla is ensconced within a supportive extracellular matrix rich in reticular fibers, collagen, and proteoglycans. These structural elements provide mechanical support and maintain the three-dimensional integrity of the adrenal medulla. Moreover, the extracellular matrix serves as a reservoir for growth factors, cytokines, and signaling molecules that modulate chromaffin cell function and plasticity. Interactions between chromaffin cells and the extracellular matrix contribute to the dynamic regulation of hormone secretion and cellular homeostasis within the adrenal medulla.

The anatomy and structure of the adrenal medulla epitomize the remarkable intricacy and functional specialization of this pivotal endocrine organ. From its embryological origins to its microscopic architecture and neural innervation, each facet of the adrenal medulla's anatomy serves a crucial role in orchestrating the body's response to stress and maintaining physiological homeostasis. A deeper understanding of the adrenal medulla's anatomy not only enriches our comprehension of endocrine physiology but also unveils novel insights into the pathophysiology of adrenal disorders and therapeutic interventions.

9.2 Adrenaline and Noradrenaline: Synthesis, Secretion, and Regulation

Adrenaline (epinephrine) and noradrenaline (norepinephrine) are catecholamines synthesized and secreted by the adrenal medulla, playing pivotal roles in the body's response to stress and other physiological stimuli. This comprehensive exploration will delve into the intricate processes involved in the synthesis, secretion, and regulation of these hormones, shedding light on their significance in maintaining homeostasis and orchestrating adaptive responses to various challenges.

Anatomy and Structure of the Adrenal Medulla:

The adrenal medulla, located within the adrenal glands atop each kidney, consists of specialized neuroendocrine cells called chromaffin cells. These cells are derived from neural crest cells and are highly vascularized, facilitating the rapid release of catecholamines into the bloodstream. Chromaffin cells receive innervation from sympathetic preganglionic fibers of the autonomic nervous system, highlighting the close interplay between the nervous and endocrine systems in regulating adrenal medulla function.

Synthesis Pathway of Adrenaline and Noradrenaline:

The synthesis of adrenaline and noradrenaline begins with the amino acid tyrosine, obtained from the diet or synthesized from phenylalanine. Within chromaffin cells, tyrosine is converted to dopamine by the enzyme tyrosine hydroxylase, a rate-limiting step in catecholamine synthesis. Dopamine is subsequently converted to noradrenaline by the enzyme dopamine beta-hydroxylase. In some species, noradrenaline can undergo methylation by phenylethanolamine N-methyltransferase (PNMT) to form adrenaline. This enzymatic cascade ensures the production of both adrenaline and noradrenaline, which serve distinct physiological roles in the body.

Secretion Mechanism of Adrenaline and Noradrenaline:

The release of adrenaline and noradrenaline from chromaffin cells is orchestrated by complex signaling pathways triggered by various stimuli, including stress and sympathetic nervous system activation. Upon stimulation, sympathetic preganglionic fibers release acetylcholine at synapses with chromaffin cells, leading to membrane depolarization. This depolarization event activates voltage-gated calcium channels, allowing calcium ions to enter the cell. Elevated intracellular calcium concentrations then facilitate the fusion of catecholamine-containing vesicles with the cell membrane, leading to the exocytotic release of adrenaline and noradrenaline into the bloodstream. This process ensures the rapid dissemination of catecholamines throughout the body, priming it for the "fight or flight" response.

Regulation of Synthesis and Secretion:

The synthesis and secretion of adrenaline and noradrenaline are subject to tight regulation by neural, hormonal, and environmental factors. Sympathetic nervous system activity plays a central role in modulating adrenal medulla function, with sympathetic nerve impulses triggering catecholamine release in response to stressors. Additionally, hormonal factors such as corticotropin-releasing hormone (CRH) and adrenocorticotropic hormone (ACTH), part of the hypothalamic-pituitary-adrenal (HPA) axis, can influence adrenal medulla activity indirectly. Furthermore, feedback mechanisms, including negative feedback loops, help maintain homeostasis by regulating the duration and intensity of the stress response. Dysregulation of these regulatory mechanisms can lead to pathological conditions such as hypertension, anxiety disorders, and pheochromocytoma, underscoring the importance of finely tuned catecholamine synthesis and secretion.

Physiological Effects of Adrenaline and Noradrenaline:

Adrenaline and noradrenaline exert profound effects on multiple organ systems, coordinating the body's physiological responses to stress and other stimuli. These effects include:

- Cardiovascular effects: Increased heart rate, cardiac output, and vasoconstriction in non-essential organs, redirecting blood flow to vital organs such as the heart and brain.

- Respiratory effects: Dilation of airways and increased respiratory rate, enhancing oxygen uptake and delivery to tissues.

- Metabolic effects: Mobilization of glucose and fatty acids from stores, providing energy substrates for increased metabolic demands during stress.

- Central nervous system effects: Heightened alertness, increased mental focus, and pupil dilation, optimizing sensory perception and cognitive function.

- Thermoregulatory effects: Increased heat production and redistribution of blood flow to maintain body temperature in response to cold stress.

- Smooth muscle effects: Relaxation of gastrointestinal smooth muscle and contraction of sphincters, diverting blood flow away from the digestive tract during the stress response.

In Summary Adrenaline and noradrenaline, synthesized and secreted by the adrenal medulla, are pivotal mediators of the body's response to stress and physiological stimuli. Through a complex interplay of synthesis, secretion, and regulation, these catecholamines orchestrate adaptive physiological responses that enable the body to cope with challenges and maintain homeostasis. A comprehensive understanding of the synthesis, secretion, and physiological effects of adrenaline and noradrenaline provides insights into their fundamental roles in health and disease, highlighting their significance in human physiology.

9.3 Functions of Adrenal Medulla Hormones: Adrenaline and Noradrenaline

These catecholamines, released in response to stress and other physiological stimuli, orchestrate a myriad of responses throughout the body, ensuring adaptive changes necessary for survival and homeostasis. This comprehensive guide aims to provide an in-depth exploration of the multifaceted functions of adrenaline and noradrenaline, delving into their cardiovascular, respiratory, metabolic, central nervous system, and endocrine effects.

Cardiovascular Effects of Adrenal Medulla Hormones:

The cardiovascular effects of adrenaline and noradrenaline are pivotal for maintaining hemodynamic stability and optimizing tissue perfusion during stress and physical exertion. By binding to adrenergic receptors on cardiac myocytes, these hormones increase heart rate (positive chronotropic effect) and contractility (positive inotropic effect), resulting in enhanced cardiac output and systemic blood pressure. Simultaneously, adrenaline and noradrenaline induce vasoconstriction in peripheral blood vessels via activation of alpha-adrenergic receptors, directing blood flow towards vital organs such as the heart, brain, and skeletal muscles. This selective redistribution of blood flow ensures efficient oxygen and nutrient delivery to tissues with heightened metabolic demands while preserving perfusion pressure. Additionally, catecholamines enhance venous return to the heart by constricting venous capacitance vessels, further augmenting cardiac preload and stroke volume. Collectively, these cardiovascular adjustments enable the body to meet increased metabolic demands and sustain physiological function during times of heightened activity or stress.

Respiratory Effects of Adrenal Medulla Hormones:

Adrenaline and noradrenaline play crucial roles in modulating respiratory function to optimize oxygen uptake and gas exchange in the lungs. Through activation of beta-adrenergic receptors on bronchial smooth muscle cells, these hormones induce bronchodilation—the widening of the airways—facilitating increased airflow and improved ventilation. This bronchodilatory response enhances oxygen delivery to alveoli and enhances carbon dioxide elimination, ensuring efficient gas exchange during periods of increased respiratory demand. Moreover, sympathetic activation triggered by adrenaline and noradrenaline results in an elevation in respiratory rate (tachypnea), further enhancing pulmonary ventilation and supporting adequate oxygenation of arterial blood. These respiratory adjustments are integral components of the body's stress response, enabling rapid adaptation to changing environmental conditions or physiological demands.

Metabolic Effects of Adrenal Medulla Hormones:

Adrenaline and noradrenaline mobilize energy reserves and regulate glucose metabolism to meet increased metabolic demands during stress and physical activity. These hormones promote glycogenolysis—the breakdown of glycogen to glucose—in the liver and skeletal muscles through activation of beta-adrenergic receptors. By stimulating the enzymatic cascade responsible for glycogen breakdown, adrenaline and noradrenaline release glucose into the bloodstream, providing an immediate source of energy for tissues. Additionally, catecholamines enhance lipolysis—the hydrolysis of triglycerides into fatty acids and glycerol—in adipose tissue, releasing free fatty acids for oxidation and energy production. Furthermore, adrenaline stimulates gluconeogenesis—the synthesis of glucose from non-carbohydrate precursors—in the liver, ensuring a continuous supply of glucose to support metabolic needs. By mobilizing glucose and fatty acids, adrenaline and noradrenaline help sustain energy production and maintain blood glucose levels within the physiological range, thereby supporting overall metabolic homeostasis during stressful conditions.

Effects on Blood Flow Distribution:

The redistribution of blood flow is a critical adaptive response during stress, ensuring optimal delivery of oxygen and nutrients to tissues with the greatest metabolic demands. Adrenaline and noradrenaline play key roles in modulating blood flow distribution by inducing vasoconstriction in non-essential organs and vasodilation in vital organs involved in the stress response. Through activation of alpha-adrenergic receptors, these hormones cause vasoconstriction in peripheral blood vessels supplying tissues such as the skin, gastrointestinal tract, and kidneys, thereby redirecting blood flow away from non-essential areas. Conversely, adrenaline and noradrenaline promote vasodilation in blood vessels supplying skeletal muscles and the brain by activating beta-adrenergic receptors, facilitating increased perfusion to these metabolically active tissues.

This selective redistribution of blood flow ensures efficient oxygen and nutrient delivery to tissues involved in the stress response or physical activity, optimizing overall physiological function and performance.

Pupillary and Central Nervous System Effects:

In addition to their cardiovascular, respiratory, and metabolic effects, adrenaline and noradrenaline exert notable influences on pupillary diameter and central nervous system function. Adrenaline stimulates the dilation of the pupils (mydriasis) by acting on alpha-adrenergic receptors in the iris dilator muscle, enhancing visual acuity and peripheral vision. This pupillary response is adaptive in situations requiring heightened alertness and visual perception, such as during stress or exposure to potential threats. Moreover, both adrenaline and noradrenaline enhance mental alertness, arousal, and vigilance by acting on central nervous system receptors, including those within the brainstem and cerebral cortex. By increasing neuronal excitability and facilitating neurotransmitter release, these hormones promote rapid cognitive and behavioral responses to environmental stimuli, enabling individuals to effectively assess and navigate challenging situations. Overall, the pupillary and central nervous system effects of adrenaline and noradrenaline contribute to the adaptive readiness of the organism to respond to stressors and maintain situational awareness.

Glycogenolysis and Gluconeogenesis:

Adrenaline and noradrenaline play pivotal roles in mobilizing glucose from hepatic glycogen stores and promoting gluconeogenesis to ensure an adequate supply of energy substrates during stress. Upon activation of beta-adrenergic receptors in hepatocytes, these hormones initiate glycogenolysis—the enzymatic breakdown of glycogen to glucose-1-phosphate and subsequently to glucose-6-phosphate. Glucose-6-phosphate can then be further processed and released into the bloodstream to maintain blood glucose levels during periods of increased demand. Additionally, adrenaline stimulates gluconeogenesis—the synthesis of glucose from non-carbohydrate precursors such as lactate, glycerol, and amino acids—in the liver. Through activation of key enzymes involved in gluconeogenesis, including phosphoenolpyruvate carboxykinase (PEPCK) and glucose-6-phosphatase, adrenaline facilitates the conversion of these substrates into glucose, which can be released into circulation to support metabolic needs. By promoting both glycogenolysis and gluconeogenesis, adrenaline and noradrenaline ensure a continuous supply of glucose to fuel essential metabolic processes and maintain energy homeostasis during periods of stress or prolonged exertion. These metabolic adaptations are essential for supporting physiological function and promoting survival in challenging environments.

9.4 Regulation of Adrenal Medulla Hormone Secretion: A Comprehensive Overview

The adrenal medulla, an integral component of the adrenal glands, plays a pivotal role in the body's response to stress. The synthesis and secretion of catecholamines, primarily adrenaline (epinephrine) and noradrenaline (norepinephrine), by chromaffin cells within the adrenal medulla are crucial for orchestrating the physiological changes necessary for adaptation and survival in challenging situations. This comprehensive review aims to delve deeply into the intricate regulatory mechanisms governing adrenal medulla hormone secretion, encompassing neural, hormonal, and feedback pathways.

Neural Regulation of Adrenal Medulla Hormone Secretion:

The sympathetic division of the autonomic nervous system serves as the primary regulator of adrenal medulla activity. Upon encountering stressors such as physical exertion, emotional stress, or environmental threats, sympathetic preganglionic fibers release acetylcholine at synapses with chromaffin cells. This neurotransmitter binds to nicotinic receptors on the chromaffin cells, triggering the depolarization of the cell membrane and the influx of calcium ions. Subsequently, calcium ions stimulate the fusion of catecholamine-containing vesicles with the cell membrane, facilitating the release of adrenaline and noradrenaline into the bloodstream. The intensity and duration of sympathetic nerve stimulation are finely tuned to match the perceived threat and ensure an appropriate stress response.

Neural Inputs Modulating Adrenal Medulla Activity:

Beyond direct sympathetic innervation, neural inputs from higher brain centers, particularly the hypothalamus, exert modulatory effects on adrenal medulla function. The hypothalamus, serving as the central integrative center for stress responses, integrates sensory information and initiates appropriate autonomic and endocrine responses through direct and indirect pathways. Neurons within the hypothalamic paraventricular nucleus (PVN) release corticotropin-releasing hormone (CRH) in response to stress signals, which stimulates the secretion of adrenocorticotropic hormone (ACTH) from the anterior pituitary gland. While ACTH primarily targets the adrenal cortex, it can also influence the adrenal medulla indirectly, albeit to a lesser extent. Additionally, inputs from other brain regions, such as the limbic system and brainstem nuclei, modulate adrenal medulla activity in response to emotional and physiological stressors, further fine-tuning the stress response.

Hormonal Regulation of Adrenal Medulla Hormone Secretion:

While neural inputs dominate the acute regulation of adrenal medulla hormone secretion, hormonal factors also play a significant role, particularly in modulating the long-term adaptive response to stress. The hypothalamic-pituitary-adrenal (HPA) axis, a key neuroendocrine system involved in stress regulation, coordinates the release of CRH and ACTH in response to stressors. CRH, synthesized and released by the hypothalamus, stimulates the anterior pituitary gland to secrete ACTH into the bloodstream. ACTH, in turn, acts on the adrenal cortex, promoting the synthesis and secretion of glucocorticoids, such as cortisol. While glucocorticoids primarily exert metabolic effects, they can also modulate adrenal medulla activity by influencing the expression of enzymes involved in catecholamine synthesis and secretion. Moreover, other hormonal factors, including angiotensin II and thyroid hormones, may indirectly influence adrenal medulla function through their effects on sympathetic activity and chromaffin cell responsiveness.

Feedback Mechanisms in Adrenal Medulla Regulation:

Maintaining physiological homeostasis necessitates the tight regulation of adrenal medulla hormone secretion through negative feedback mechanisms. Elevated levels of circulating catecholamines can inhibit further release via negative feedback loops involving both neural and hormonal pathways. Direct effects on chromaffin cells, such as desensitization of adrenergic receptors or downregulation of catecholamine synthesis enzymes, contribute to the termination of the stress response. Additionally, feedback inhibition may involve indirect effects on regulatory centers within the central nervous system and hypothalamus, dampening sympathetic outflow and reducing CRH and ACTH secretion. These feedback loops ensure that the stress response is appropriately terminated once the stressor is no longer present, preventing excessive catecholamine release and associated adverse effects.

Circadian Regulation of Adrenal Medulla Activity:

Adrenal medulla hormone secretion exhibits diurnal variation, with peak levels occurring in the morning hours. This temporal pattern is governed by the master circadian clock located in the suprachiasmatic nucleus of the hypothalamus, which synchronizes physiological processes with the light-dark cycle. The circadian rhythm of adrenal medulla activity is influenced by both neural and hormonal inputs, with sympathetic nerve activity and glucocorticoid levels displaying rhythmic variations throughout the day. The synchronization of adrenal medulla function with the circadian rhythm ensures optimal physiological responses to stressors at different times of the day, promoting energy conservation during periods of rest and heightened alertness during the waking hours.

In summary the regulation of adrenal medulla hormone secretion involves a complex interplay of neural, hormonal, and feedback mechanisms, finely tuned to match the intensity and duration of stressors encountered by the organism. Neural inputs from the sympathetic nervous system and higher brain centers coordinate the acute stress response, while hormonal factors, including those from the HPA axis, modulate the long-term adaptive response to stress. Negative feedback mechanisms ensure the termination of the stress response once the stressor is removed, preventing excessive catecholamine release. Furthermore, the circadian regulation of adrenal medulla activity ensures temporal coordination of physiological processes with the daily light-dark cycle.

Case Studies

Case Study 1: Pheochromocytoma and Catecholamine Hypersecretion

Patient Profile:

- Name: Mary Johnson

- Age: 50 years

- Sex: Female

- Occupation: Teacher

- Medical History: Hypertension, anxiety

- Family History: Father had hypertension and heart disease

Presentation:

Mary presents with episodic symptoms of severe headaches, palpitations, sweating, and high blood pressure spikes. These episodes last for about 15-20 minutes and occur several times a week. She also reports feeling extremely anxious and having trouble sleeping.

Physical Examination:

- Vital Signs: BP: 180/110 mmHg, HR: 95 bpm, Temp: 37.0°C

- General Appearance: Anxious and diaphoretic

- Cardiovascular Examination: No abnormalities detected

- Endocrine Examination: Normal

Laboratory Tests:

- Plasma Metanephrines: Elevated

- 24-Hour Urinary Catecholamines: Elevated

- CT Scan of Abdomen: Adrenal mass detected

Discussion:

Mary's symptoms and test results suggest a pheochromocytoma, a rare tumor of the adrenal medulla that results in excessive production of catecholamines (epinephrine and norepinephrine). This condition leads to episodic hypertension and other related symptoms.

Questions:

1. Explain the role of the adrenal medulla in the production of catecholamines.

2. Discuss the physiological effects of epinephrine and norepinephrine.

3. How do catecholamines regulate cardiovascular function?

4. Describe the feedback mechanism involved in catecholamine regulation.

Case Study 2: Chronic Stress and Adrenal Medulla Hyperactivity

Patient Profile:

- Name: John Smith

- Age: 40 years

- Sex: Male

- Occupation: IT Manager

- Medical History: No significant past medical history

- Family History: Mother has diabetes type 2

Presentation:

John reports experiencing chronic stress due to work pressures. He mentions symptoms such as constant fatigue, difficulty concentrating, and frequent episodes of rapid heart rate and sweating. He also reports poor sleep quality and irritability.

Physical Examination:

- Vital Signs: BP: 135/85 mmHg, HR: 90 bpm, Temp: 36.7°C

- General Appearance: Appears tired and stressed

- Cardiovascular Examination: No abnormalities detected

- Endocrine Examination: Normal

Laboratory Tests:

- Plasma Catecholamines: Moderately elevated

- Cortisol (Morning): Elevated

- ACTH (Adrenocorticotropic Hormone): Normal

Discussion:

John's symptoms and lab results indicate chronic stress, leading to hyperactivity of the adrenal medulla. The elevated catecholamines and cortisol suggest an ongoing stress response, affecting his overall well-being and health.

Questions:

1. Describe the role of the adrenal medulla in the stress response.

2. What are the effects of chronic elevation of catecholamines on the body?

3. Explain the interaction between the adrenal medulla and the HPA axis during stress.

4. How can chronic stress impact long-term health?

Practice Questions for Self-Assessment

Multiple Choice Questions

1. Which of the following hormones is primarily produced by the adrenal medulla?

   a) Cortisol

   b) Aldosterone

   c) Epinephrine

   d) Insulin

2. The primary function of catecholamines during the fight-or-flight response is to:

   a) Decrease heart rate

   b) Increase blood glucose levels

   c) Reduce blood pressure

   d) Promote digestion

3. Pheochromocytoma is a tumor of which part of the adrenal gland?

   a) Adrenal cortex

   b) Adrenal medulla

   c) Zona glomerulosa

   d) Zona fasciculata

4. The secretion of catecholamines from the adrenal medulla is directly stimulated by:

   a) ACTH

   b) CRH

c) Sympathetic nervous system

d) Parasympathetic nervous system

5. Which enzyme is responsible for the conversion of norepinephrine to epinephrine in the adrenal medulla?

a) Tyrosine hydroxylase

b) Dopamine β-hydroxylase

c) Phenylethanolamine N-methyltransferase (PNMT)

d) Monoamine oxidase

Short Answer Questions

1. Describe the biosynthetic pathway of catecholamines in the adrenal medulla.

2. Explain the role of epinephrine in the regulation of metabolism.

3. Discuss how the adrenal medulla interacts with the sympathetic nervous system.

4. Describe the physiological effects of catecholamines on the cardiovascular system.

5. Explain the potential health consequences of long-term elevated catecholamine levels.

True or False Questions

1. The adrenal medulla primarily secretes steroid hormones. (True/False)

2. Catecholamines are derived from the amino acid tyrosine. (True/False)

3. Epinephrine decreases blood glucose levels. (True/False)

4. The adrenal medulla responds to sympathetic nervous system activation. (True/False)

5. Pheochromocytoma can cause episodic hypertension. (True/False)

Answers

Case Study 1

1. Roe of Adrenal Medulla in Catecholamine Production:

   - The adrenal medulla produces catecholamines (epinephrine and norepinephrine) from the amino acid tyrosine. These hormones are stored in chromaffin cells and released into the bloodstream in response to stress signals from the sympathetic nervous system.

2. Physiological Effects of Epinephrine and Norepinephrine:

   - Epinephrine and norepinephrine increase heart rate, contractility, and blood pressure, dilate airways, and mobilize energy by increasing blood glucose and fatty acid levels. They prepare the body for a "fight-or-flight" response.

3. Catecholamines and Cardiovascular Function:

   - Catecholamines enhance cardiovascular function by increasing cardiac output and redistributing blood to essential organs like the heart and muscles. They cause vasoconstriction in non-essential areas, raising blood pressure.

4. Feedback Mechanism in Catecholamine Regulation:

   - Catecholamine release is primarily regulated by the autonomic nervous system rather than a classic feedback loop. Stress and physical activity stimulate the sympathetic nervous system, triggering catecholamine release. The resulting physiological changes help manage the stressor and restore homeostasis.

Case Study 2

1. Role of Adrenal Medulla in Stress Response:

   - The adrenal medulla is part of the sympathetic-adrenal-medullary (SAM) system, which activates during stress. It releases catecholamines, preparing the body for immediate physical activity by increasing heart rate, blood pressure, and energy availability.

2. Effects of Chronic Elevation of Catecholamines:

- Chronic elevation of catecholamines can lead to hypertension, increased risk of cardiovascular diseases, impaired glucose metabolism, anxiety, and other stress-related disorders.

3. Interaction Between Adrenal Medulla and HPA Axis:

- During stress, the HPA axis releases cortisol, which has a slower and prolonged effect. The adrenal medulla's catecholamines provide immediate response. Together, they coordinate to manage acute and chronic stress.

4. Impact of Chronic Stress on Health:

- Chronic stress can lead to sustained high levels of catecholamines and cortisol, causing immune suppression, cardiovascular diseases, metabolic disorders, mental health issues, and other health problems.

Multiple Choice Questions

1. c) Epinephrine

2. b) Increase blood glucose levels

3. b) Adrenal medulla

4. c) Sympathetic nervous system

5. c) Phenylethanolamine N-methyltransferase (PNMT)

Short Answer Questions

1. Biosynthetic Pathway of Catecholamines:

- Catecholamines are synthesized from tyrosine. Tyrosine is converted to DOPA by tyrosine hydroxylase, then to dopamine by DOPA decarboxylase. Dopamine is converted to norepinephrine by dopamine β-hydroxylase, and finally, norepinephrine is converted to epinephrine by phenylethanolamine N-methyltransferase (PNMT).

2. Role of Epinephrine in Metabolism:

- Epinephrine increases glycogenolysis in the liver and muscle, promotes lipolysis in adipose tissue, and inhibits insulin secretion, all of which increase blood glucose and fatty acid levels to provide energy during stress.

3. Adrenal Medulla and Sympathetic Nervous System:

   - The adrenal medulla acts as an extension of the sympathetic nervous system. It releases catecholamines in response to sympathetic stimulation, amplifying and prolonging the effects of sympathetic activation throughout the body.

4. Effects of Catecholamines on Cardiovascular System:

   - Catecholamines increase heart rate, myocardial contractility, and conduction velocity. They cause vasoconstriction in peripheral blood vessels and vasodilation in skeletal muscles, enhancing blood flow to vital organs during stress.

5. Health Consequences of Long-term Elevated Catecholamine Levels:

   - Prolonged high catecholamine levels can lead to chronic hypertension, increased risk of heart disease, metabolic disturbances, anxiety, insomnia, and other stress-related conditions.

True or False Questions

1. False

2. True

3. False

4. True

5. True

Bibliography

1. Axelrod, J. (1976). The pineal gland: A neurochemical transducer. Science, 184(4135), 134-143.

   - This classic paper discusses the neurochemical role of the pineal gland and provides context for understanding the function of the adrenal medulla in neuroendocrine systems.

2. Cannon, W. B. (1939). The Wisdom of the Body. W.W. Norton & Company.

   - Cannon's work introduces the concept of homeostasis and the role of the adrenal medulla in the 'fight or flight' response, foundational knowledge for understanding adrenal medulla physiology.

3. Eisenhofer, G., Goldstein, D. S., & Kopin, I. J. (2004). Catecholamine metabolism: A contemporary view with implications for physiology and medicine. Pharmacological Reviews, 56(3), 331-349.

   - This review article provides a comprehensive overview of catecholamine metabolism, highlighting the adrenal medulla's role in synthesizing adrenaline and noradrenaline.

4. Gore, A. C. (Ed.). (2010). Endocrine-Disrupting Chemicals: From Basic Research to Clinical Practice. Humana Press.

   - This book covers various aspects of endocrine disruption, including how certain chemicals can affect adrenal medulla function and hormone secretion.

5. Kvetnansky, R., Sabban, E. L., & Palkovits, M. (2009). Catecholaminergic systems in stress: Structural and molecular genetic approaches. Physiological Reviews, 89(2), 535-606.

   - This article explores the role of catecholamines in stress responses, with a focus on the adrenal medulla's function in producing these crucial hormones.

6. Landsberg, L., & Young, J. B. (1978). Fasting, feeding and regulation of the sympathetic nervous system. New England Journal of Medicine, 298(23), 1295-1301.

   - This paper investigates the relationship between metabolic states and sympathetic nervous system activity, pertinent to understanding how the adrenal medulla regulates energy balance.

7. Pacak, K., & Eisenhofer, G. (2007). An overview of the adrenal medulla: Physiology, histology, and regulation. In Pheochromocytoma: Diagnosis, Localization, and Treatment (pp. 7-33). Humana Press.

   - This book chapter provides a detailed overview of the adrenal medulla's anatomy, hormone synthesis, and regulatory mechanisms.

8. Schultz, R. A., & Beaven, M. A. (1980). Catecholamines and Their Receptors in the Adrenal Medulla. Biochemical Pharmacology, 29(21), 2991-2997.

- This paper discusses the biochemical pathways involved in catecholamine synthesis and the receptor interactions critical to adrenal medulla function.

9. Silva, P. (Ed.). (2011). Textbook of Physiology. Elsevier Health Sciences.

- This textbook covers the physiological aspects of the adrenal medulla, including its role in homeostasis and response to stress.

10. Vinson, G. P. (2009). The Adrenal Cortex and Life: Selected studies in structure and function. Springer Science & Business Media.

- While primarily focused on the adrenal cortex, this book also provides relevant insights into the adrenal medulla's interaction with cortical hormones and overall adrenal function.

Chapter 10

Physiology of Endocrine Pancreas and Glucose Metabolism

The endocrine pancreas, comprising the islets of Langerhans, plays a critical role in regulating blood glucose levels and metabolic homeostasis. This chapter explores the physiology of the endocrine pancreas, focusing on the synthesis, secretion, and actions of insulin and glucagon, as well as the intricate mechanisms involved in glucose metabolism.

10.1 Islets of Langerhans: Composition and Functions:

The islets of Langerhans, nestled within the pancreas, serve as the orchestrators of metabolic symphony, finely tuning blood glucose levels and maintaining metabolic equilibrium. Despite constituting only a fraction of the pancreatic tissue, these microorgans play an outsized role in regulating glucose metabolism and hormone secretion. Let's delve deeper into the intricate composition and multifaceted functions of the islets of Langerhans.

Composition of Islets of Langerhans

Within the labyrinthine architecture of the pancreas, the islets of Langerhans emerge as discrete clusters of cells, each contributing distinctively to the metabolic orchestra:

1. Beta Cells:

   At the heart of the islets lie the beta cells, the virtuosos of insulin production. These cells, comprising the majority of the islet population, choreograph the release of insulin in response to the crescendo of rising blood glucose levels. Through their meticulous synthesis and secretion of insulin, beta cells regulate glucose uptake by peripheral tissues, promoting cellular glucose uptake, glycogen synthesis, and lipogenesis.

2. Alpha Cells:

   In counterpoint to the beta cells, the alpha cells resonate with the rhythm of glucagon. Occupying a notable fraction of the islet milieu, these cells sense the ebb of blood glucose levels and respond by releasing glucagon. This hormone acts as a symphony conductor, orchestrating the release of glucose from hepatic glycogen stores through glycogenolysis and stimulating gluconeogenesis, thus elevating blood glucose levels to meet metabolic demands.

3. Delta Cells:

Interspersed among the beta and alpha cells, the delta cells stand as sentinels of metabolic equilibrium. They synthesize and release somatostatin, a paracrine and endocrine regulator that modulates the secretion of both insulin and glucagon. Through its inhibitory effects on hormone release, somatostatin harmonizes the interplay between insulin and glucagon, ensuring precise control over blood glucose levels.

4. Pancreatic Polypeptide (PP) Cells:

A lesser-known troupe within the islets, the pancreatic polypeptide (PP) cells contribute to the regulation of exocrine pancreatic function and appetite regulation. By secreting pancreatic polypeptide, these cells fine-tune the pancreatic digestive enzyme secretion and influence satiety signals, thereby modulating food intake and energy balance.

5. Epsilon Cells:

Lastly, the epsilon cells, though sparse in number, resonate with the rhythm of hunger and satiety. They secrete ghrelin, a hormone that signals hunger and stimulates appetite. Ghrelin levels rise during fasting periods, signaling the brain to initiate feeding behaviors, thus playing a crucial role in the regulation of energy balance and metabolic homeostasis.

Functions of Islets of Langerhans

Within the bustling microcosm of the islets of Langerhans, a symphony of metabolic processes unfolds:

1. Glucose Sensing and Hormone Secretion:

The beta cells, finely attuned to the flux of blood glucose levels, modulate their insulin secretion accordingly. Elevated glucose levels stimulate insulin release, while decreased levels inhibit its secretion. Conversely, alpha cells respond to low glucose levels by secreting glucagon, thus initiating a cascade of events aimed at restoring euglycemia.

2. Integration of Metabolic Signals:

Islet cells serve as metabolic maestros, integrating diverse signals such as glucose, amino acids, fatty acids, and neural inputs to regulate hormone secretion. Incretin hormones released from the gut in response to nutrient ingestion amplify insulin secretion, ensuring an appropriate response to nutrient intake.

3. Metabolic Adaptation:

Islet cells exhibit remarkable plasticity, adjusting their function in response to fluctuating metabolic demands. During fasting or exercise, glucagon predominates, mobilizing stored energy reserves to sustain metabolic needs. Conversely, postprandial periods are characterized by increased insulin secretion to facilitate nutrient uptake and storage.

4. Regulation of Hormone Interactions:

Somatostatin emerges as the conductor of hormonal harmony within the islets, fine-tuning the balance between insulin and glucagon secretion. By exerting inhibitory effects on both hormones, somatostatin ensures precise control over blood glucose levels and prevents erratic fluctuations.

Clinical Implications and Pathophysiology

Understanding the nuances of islet cell composition and function has profound clinical implications, particularly in the realm of metabolic disorders such as diabetes mellitus:

1. Type 1 Diabetes:

Autoimmune destruction of beta cells leads to absolute insulin deficiency in type 1 diabetes. Consequently, individuals with this condition require exogenous insulin therapy to maintain glycemic control and prevent acute and chronic complications.

2. Type 2 Diabetes:

In type 2 diabetes, a combination of insulin resistance and relative insulin deficiency contributes to hyperglycemia. Dysfunction of beta cells, coupled with impaired insulin action, necessitates comprehensive management strategies encompassing lifestyle modifications, oral medications, and, in some cases, insulin therapy.

3. Islet Transplantation:

Islet transplantation holds promise as a therapeutic modality for type 1 diabetes, aiming to restore beta cell function and achieve insulin independence. Advances in islet isolation techniques and immunosuppressive protocols have fueled optimism regarding the long-term efficacy of this approach.

4. Future Therapeutic Strategies:

Ongoing research endeavors focused on unraveling the molecular intricacies of islet cell function may yield novel therapeutic targets for diabetes management. Strategies aimed at preserving or restoring beta cell mass and function represent promising avenues for future intervention.

10.2 Insulin: Synthesis, Secretion, and Actions

Insulin, a peptide hormone synthesized and secreted by the beta cells of the pancreatic islets of Langerhans, is a key regulator of glucose metabolism and plays a central role in maintaining blood glucose homeostasis. Its synthesis, secretion, and actions are intricately orchestrated to respond dynamically to changes in nutrient availability and metabolic demands. This section provides an in-depth exploration of the processes involved in the synthesis, secretion, and diverse actions of insulin.

Synthesis of Insulin:

Insulin synthesis is a highly regulated process that occurs within the endoplasmic reticulum (ER) and Golgi apparatus of beta cells. The journey of insulin synthesis begins with the transcription of the insulin gene (INS) into preproinsulin, a single polypeptide chain consisting of a signal peptide, A chain, B chain, and connecting C-peptide. This precursor molecule, preproinsulin, is then translocated into the ER, where the signal peptide is cleaved, yielding proinsulin.

Within the ER, proinsulin undergoes folding and disulfide bond formation, facilitated by chaperone proteins, to attain its native conformation. Proinsulin is then transported to the Golgi apparatus, where it is packaged into secretory vesicles called granules. Within these granules, proinsulin is processed further by proteolytic enzymes known as prohormone convertases, which cleave the connecting C-peptide, resulting in the formation of mature insulin and C-peptide.

The mature insulin molecules are stored within secretory granules, ready for release in response to physiological stimuli. The presence of both insulin and C-peptide in equimolar amounts within secretory granules serves as a marker of beta cell function and provides insight into insulin secretion dynamics.

Secretion of Insulin:

Insulin secretion is tightly regulated by multiple factors, including blood glucose levels, amino acids, gastrointestinal hormones, neural inputs, and metabolic hormones. The primary stimulus for insulin secretion is elevated blood glucose levels, which trigger a series of events culminating in the release of insulin from beta cells.

In response to increased blood glucose concentrations, glucose enters beta cells via the facilitated glucose transporter GLUT2. Within the cytoplasm, glucose undergoes glycolysis, leading to the generation of ATP. The resulting increase in the ATP/ADP ratio leads to the closure of ATP-sensitive potassium (KATP) channels, causing membrane depolarization.

Membrane depolarization triggers the opening of voltage-gated calcium channels, allowing calcium ions to influx into the cell. The rise in intracellular calcium levels triggers exocytosis of insulin-containing vesicles, resulting in the release of insulin into the bloodstream. This process, known as exocytosis, is finely tuned to ensure rapid and precise control of insulin secretion in response to fluctuations in blood glucose levels.

In addition to glucose, other nutrients such as amino acids, particularly leucine and arginine, stimulate insulin secretion through mechanisms involving mitochondrial metabolism and ATP production. Gastrointestinal hormones such as incretins (e.g., glucagon-like peptide-1 or GLP-1) released in response to food intake potentiate glucose-stimulated insulin secretion, a phenomenon known as the incretin effect.

Neural inputs from the autonomic nervous system, including both sympathetic and parasympathetic pathways, also modulate insulin secretion. Sympathetic stimulation inhibits insulin secretion, whereas parasympathetic stimulation enhances it, reflecting the body's integrated response to stress and metabolic demands.

Furthermore, metabolic hormones such as glucagon, cortisol, and catecholamines exert regulatory effects on insulin secretion, modulating pancreatic beta cell function in response to fasting, stress, and other physiological challenges.

Actions of Insulin:

Insulin exerts a broad spectrum of metabolic and regulatory effects on target tissues throughout the body, coordinating glucose uptake, utilization, and storage to maintain metabolic homeostasis. The actions of insulin can be categorized into several key physiological processes:

1. Glucose Uptake:

Insulin facilitates the uptake of glucose into insulin-sensitive tissues, including skeletal muscle, adipose tissue, and the liver, by promoting the translocation of glucose transporters (GLUT4) to the cell membrane. In skeletal muscle and adipose tissue, insulin binding to its receptor initiates a cascade of intracellular signaling events that culminate in the translocation of GLUT4-containing vesicles to the cell surface, increasing glucose uptake.

2. Glycogen Synthesis:

Insulin promotes glycogen synthesis (glycogenesis) in the liver and skeletal muscle by activating glycogen synthase and inhibiting glycogen phosphorylase, key enzymes involved in glycogen metabolism. This process allows excess glucose to be stored in the form of glycogen for future use, preventing hyperglycemia and providing a readily available energy source during times of need.

3. Inhibition of Gluconeogenesis:

Insulin suppresses hepatic gluconeogenesis, the process by which the liver produces glucose from non-carbohydrate precursors such as lactate, amino acids, and glycerol. Insulin exerts inhibitory effects on key enzymes involved in gluconeogenesis, including phosphoenolpyruvate carboxykinase (PEPCK) and glucose-6-phosphatase (G6Pase), thereby reducing the production of glucose and contributing to the maintenance of euglycemia.

4. Protein Synthesis:

Insulin promotes protein synthesis and inhibits protein degradation, particularly in skeletal muscle. By stimulating the uptake of amino acids into cells and activating key signaling pathways involved in protein synthesis (e.g., mTOR pathway), insulin facilitates the assembly of new proteins, contributing to tissue growth, repair, and maintenance.

5. Lipid Metabolism:

Insulin regulates lipid metabolism by promoting lipogenesis (the synthesis of fatty acids and triglycerides) and inhibiting lipolysis (the breakdown of triglycerides into fatty acids) in adipose tissue. In the presence of insulin, adipocytes take up glucose and convert it into glycerol-3-phosphate, a precursor for triglyceride synthesis, while fatty acid synthesis is stimulated by the conversion of excess glucose and amino acids into acetyl-CoA.

6. Cellular Growth and Differentiation:

Insulin exerts mitogenic effects on various cell types, including hepatocytes, adipocytes, and vascular endothelial cells, promoting cell growth, proliferation, and differentiation. Through activation of growth-promoting signaling pathways such as the MAPK/ERK pathway and PI3K/Akt pathway, insulin stimulates cell cycle progression and cellular hypertrophy, contributing to tissue development and homeostasis.

7. Regulation of Ion Transport:

Insulin modulates ion transport across cell membranes, influencing the movement of potassium, magnesium, and phosphate ions in various tissues. By promoting potassium uptake and intracellular retention, insulin contributes to the maintenance of cellular membrane potential and electrolyte balance, essential for normal cellular function and excitability.

Clinical Relevance:

Dysfunction in insulin synthesis, secretion, or action can lead to metabolic disorders such as diabetes mellitus, characterized by impaired glucose homeostasis and dysregulated metabolism. Type 1 diabetes mellitus results from autoimmune destruction of pancreatic beta cells, leading to absolute insulin deficiency and dependence on exogenous insulin replacement therapy.

In contrast, type 2 diabetes mellitus is characterized by insulin resistance, impaired insulin secretion, and dysregulated hepatic glucose production, often in the context of obesity and metabolic syndrome. Therapeutic interventions for diabetes aim to restore insulin function, either by providing exogenous insulin (insulin replacement therapy) or by targeting insulin resistance and secretion defects with oral antidiabetic medications, injectable incretin-based therapies, and other pharmacological agents.

A deeper understanding of the synthesis, secretion, and actions of insulin is essential for elucidating the pathophysiology of diabetes and developing targeted therapeutic strategies to manage this complex metabolic disorder effectively.

In conclusion, insulin serves as a master regulator of glucose metabolism and exerts a myriad of metabolic, growth-promoting, and regulatory effects on target tissues throughout the body. Its synthesis, secretion, and actions are tightly regulated to maintain metabolic homeostasis and respond adaptively to changes in nutrient availability and physiological demands. By unraveling the intricacies of insulin biology, researchers continue to uncover new insights into the pathogenesis of diabetes and explore innovative approaches for its prevention and treatment.

10.3 Glucagon: Synthesis, Secretion, and Actions:

Glucagon, a peptide hormone produced by alpha cells within the pancreatic islets of Langerhans, serves as a vital regulator of glucose metabolism and plays a key role in maintaining blood glucose homeostasis. Its synthesis, secretion, and actions are intricately orchestrated to ensure adequate glucose availability during periods of fasting, exercise, or stress. This section provides a detailed exploration of glucagon's molecular biology, regulation, physiological effects, and clinical significance.

Synthesis and Secretion:

The synthesis of glucagon begins with the transcription of the glucagon gene (GCG) in pancreatic alpha cells. The primary transcript, preproglucagon, undergoes post-translational processing in the endoplasmic reticulum to form proglucagon. Proglucagon is then transported to the Golgi apparatus, where it is further processed by prohormone convertases (PC1/3 in alpha cells) to yield the mature hormone, glucagon. The fully processed glucagon is stored in secretory granules within the alpha cells, ready for release in response to physiological stimuli.

Glucagon secretion is tightly regulated by multiple factors, including blood glucose levels, amino acids, sympathetic nervous system activity, and hormonal signals. The primary stimulus for glucagon release is hypoglycemia, which activates alpha cells to secrete glucagon into the bloodstream. In addition to low glucose levels, sympathetic stimulation, mediated by catecholamines such as adrenaline, can also trigger glucagon secretion, providing an additional mechanism to mobilize glucose during stress or exercise. Moreover, certain amino acids, particularly alanine and arginine, stimulate glucagon secretion, reflecting the role of protein metabolism in regulating glucose homeostasis.

Actions of Glucagon:

Glucagon exerts its physiological effects through interactions with specific G protein-coupled receptors (GPCRs) expressed on target cells, primarily hepatocytes in the liver. Upon binding to its receptor, glucagon activates adenylate cyclase, leading to the production of cyclic AMP (cAMP) and activation of protein kinase A (PKA) signaling pathway. This intracellular cascade phosphorylates key enzymes and proteins involved in glucose metabolism, leading to the following actions:

1. Stimulation of Glycogenolysis: Glucagon promotes the breakdown of glycogen stored in the liver (glycogenolysis) by activating glycogen phosphorylase, the rate-limiting enzyme in glycogen degradation. Phosphorylation of glycogen phosphorylase by PKA enhances its activity, resulting in the release of glucose-1-phosphate from glycogen molecules. Glucose-1-phosphate is subsequently converted into glucose-6-phosphate, a precursor for glucose production or glycolysis, depending on the metabolic needs of the cell.

2. Promotion of Gluconeogenesis: Glucagon stimulates gluconeogenesis, the synthesis of glucose from non-carbohydrate precursors such as lactate, glycerol, and amino acids. Gluconeogenesis occurs primarily in the liver and is essential for maintaining blood glucose levels during fasting or prolonged exercise. Glucagon upregulates the expression of key enzymes involved in gluconeogenesis, including phosphoenolpyruvate carboxykinase (PEPCK) and glucose-6-phosphatase, through the activation of transcription factors such as CREB (cAMP response element-binding protein).

3. Enhancement of Lipolysis: Glucagon promotes the breakdown of triglycerides stored in adipose tissue into glycerol and free fatty acids, a process known as lipolysis. Glycerol released from adipocytes can serve as a substrate for gluconeogenesis in the liver, contributing to the maintenance of blood glucose levels during fasting or prolonged energy expenditure. Free fatty acids released into the bloodstream can be utilized as an alternative energy source by various tissues, sparing glucose for glucose-dependent organs such as the brain and red blood cells.

Regulation of Glucagon Secretion:

Glucagon secretion is subject to intricate regulation to ensure precise control over blood glucose levels in response to physiological cues. The primary determinant of glucagon secretion is the concentration of blood glucose, with low glucose levels stimulating glucagon release and high glucose levels inhibiting it through negative feedback mechanisms. Glucose sensing in alpha cells is mediated by ATP-sensitive potassium (KATP) channels, which close in response to low glucose levels, leading to membrane depolarization and calcium influx, triggering glucagon secretion. Conversely, high glucose levels lead to KATP channel opening, hyperpolarization, and suppression of glucagon release.

In addition to glucose, other factors influence glucagon secretion, including amino acids, gastrointestinal hormones, and neural inputs. Amino acids, particularly alanine and arginine, directly stimulate glucagon secretion by alpha cells, providing a link between protein metabolism and glucose homeostasis. Gastrointestinal hormones such as incretins (e.g., glucagon-like peptide-1 or GLP-1) can modulate glucagon secretion indirectly through paracrine effects on alpha cells. Furthermore, neural inputs from the autonomic nervous system, specifically sympathetic activation, can stimulate glucagon secretion during stress or exercise, mobilizing glucose reserves to meet increased metabolic demands.

Clinical Significance:

Dysregulation of glucagon secretion and signaling is implicated in the pathophysiology of various metabolic disorders, including diabetes mellitus and hypoglycemia. In type 1 diabetes mellitus, autoimmune destruction of pancreatic beta cells leads to insulin deficiency and unopposed glucagon action, resulting in unchecked hepatic glucose production and hyperglycemia. Conversely, in type 2 diabetes mellitus, impaired alpha cell function and glucagon dysregulation contribute to hyperglucagonemia and exacerbate hyperglycemia. Therapeutic interventions targeting glucagon signaling pathways are being explored as potential strategies for the management of diabetes and other metabolic disorders. Glucagon receptor antagonists, which inhibit glucagon action, have shown promise in improving glycemic control and reducing hepatic glucose production in preclinical and clinical studies.

10.4 Regulation of Blood Glucose Levels: A Comprehensive Exploration of Physiological Mechanisms and Clinical Implications:

The regulation of blood glucose levels is a fundamental aspect of metabolic homeostasis, essential for providing energy to cells and tissues throughout the body. This intricate process involves the coordinated action of hormones, neural signals, and metabolic pathways to maintain blood glucose within a narrow physiological range, ensuring optimal cellular function. In this comprehensive exploration, we will delve into the multifaceted mechanisms governing blood glucose regulation, examining the roles of insulin, glucagon, counterregulatory hormones, neural inputs, and their interplay in health and disease.

Fed State Regulation:

In the fed state, following a meal, the body experiences an influx of nutrients, including glucose, from the gastrointestinal tract. This triggers a series of metabolic responses aimed at utilizing and storing excess nutrients, particularly glucose, for future energy needs.

1. Insulin-Mediated Glucose Uptake and Utilization:

- Insulin, secreted by pancreatic beta cells in response to elevated blood glucose levels, plays a central role in promoting glucose uptake and utilization in peripheral tissues.

- Upon binding to insulin receptors on target cells, insulin stimulates the translocation of glucose transporters (GLUT4) to the cell membrane, facilitating glucose uptake into muscle, adipose tissue, and other insulin-sensitive tissues.

- In muscle cells, insulin promotes glucose utilization for energy production (glycolysis) and glycogen synthesis, contributing to muscle function and energy storage.

- Adipose tissue takes up glucose and converts it into fatty acids through lipogenesis, leading to the storage of triglycerides in adipocytes.

2. Inhibition of Hepatic Glucose Production:

- In addition to promoting glucose uptake in peripheral tissues, insulin suppresses hepatic glucose production by inhibiting gluconeogenesis and glycogenolysis in the liver.

- Insulin inhibits key enzymes involved in gluconeogenesis, such as phosphoenolpyruvate carboxykinase (PEPCK) and glucose-6-phosphatase, thereby reducing the liver's capacity to produce glucose from non-carbohydrate precursors.

- Furthermore, insulin promotes glycogen synthesis in the liver, diverting excess glucose from the bloodstream into glycogen stores for storage and future use.

Fasting State Regulation:

During fasting or periods of energy deprivation, when glucose availability decreases, the body initiates adaptive responses to maintain blood glucose levels and meet the energy demands of vital organs and tissues.

1. Glucagon-Mediated Glucose Mobilization:

- Glucagon, released by pancreatic alpha cells in response to falling blood glucose levels, promotes glucose mobilization from hepatic glycogen stores through glycogenolysis.

- Glycogen phosphorylase and other glycogenolysis enzymes are activated by glucagon, leading to the rapid breakdown of glycogen into glucose units in the liver.

- Glucagon also stimulates gluconeogenesis, the synthesis of glucose from non-carbohydrate precursors such as amino acids and glycerol, primarily in the liver.

- These gluconeogenic substrates are converted into glucose, which is released into the bloodstream to maintain blood glucose levels and meet the energy demands of peripheral tissues.

2. Lipolysis and Ketogenesis:

- In addition to promoting glucose production, glucagon enhances lipolysis, the breakdown of triglycerides into fatty acids and glycerol, primarily in adipose tissue.

- Fatty acids released during lipolysis serve as alternative energy substrates for tissues such as muscle and the heart, conserving glucose for essential organs.

- Glycerol, a byproduct of lipolysis, can be converted into glucose through gluconeogenesis, further contributing to blood glucose maintenance.

- Excessive fatty acid oxidation in the liver leads to the production of ketone bodies, such as acetoacetate and beta-hydroxybutyrate, which serve as alternative fuels for the brain and other tissues during prolonged fasting or starvation.

Counterregulatory Hormones:

In addition to insulin and glucagon, several counterregulatory hormones, including cortisol, growth hormone, and catecholamines, play pivotal roles in modulating blood glucose levels and ensuring adequate glucose supply to tissues under various physiological conditions.

1. Cortisol:

- Cortisol, the primary glucocorticoid hormone secreted by the adrenal cortex, exerts profound effects on glucose metabolism.

- During periods of stress or fasting, cortisol levels rise, promoting gluconeogenesis and glycogenolysis in the liver.

- Cortisol stimulates the transcription of key enzymes involved in gluconeogenesis, such as phosphoenolpyruvate carboxykinase (PEPCK) and glucose-6-phosphatase, enhancing glucose production.

- Additionally, cortisol antagonizes insulin action in peripheral tissues, leading to insulin resistance and decreased glucose uptake.

2. Growth Hormone (GH):

- Growth hormone, secreted by the anterior pituitary gland, plays a critical role in regulating glucose metabolism, particularly during fasting or periods of energy deprivation.

- GH promotes lipolysis in adipose tissue, releasing fatty acids into the bloodstream for use as energy substrates.

- GH also antagonizes insulin action, reducing glucose uptake in peripheral tissues and sparing glucose for essential organs such as the brain.

- Furthermore, GH stimulates hepatic gluconeogenesis, contributing to the maintenance of blood glucose levels during fasting.

3. Catecholamines (Epinephrine and Norepinephrine):

- Epinephrine and norepinephrine, secreted by the adrenal medulla in response to stress or sympathetic activation, exert potent effects on glucose metabolism.

- These catecholamines enhance hepatic glycogenolysis and gluconeogenesis, increasing blood glucose levels in response to acute stressors.

- Epinephrine and norepinephrine also promote lipolysis in adipose tissue, releasing fatty acids for energy production and conserving glucose for vital organs.

- Additionally, catecholamines stimulate glycogenolysis in skeletal muscle, providing an immediate source of glucose for muscle contraction during fight-or-flight responses.

Neural Regulation:

The autonomic nervous system, particularly the sympathetic branch, plays a crucial role in modulating glucose metabolism through its effects on insulin and glucagon secretion, as well as hepatic glucose production. Sympathetic activation, induced by stress, exercise, or hypoglycemia, can influence blood glucose levels by altering hormonal secretion and peripheral glucose uptake.

1. Sympathetic Regulation of Hormonal Secretion:

   - Sympathetic stimulation can enhance glucagon secretion from pancreatic alpha cells, promoting glucose mobilization from hepatic glycogen stores.

   - Conversely, sympathetic activation may inhibit insulin secretion from pancreatic beta cells, reducing peripheral glucose uptake and favoring glucose production.

   - These effects help ensure a rapid response to stress or energy demands by mobilizing glucose and conserving energy substrates for vital functions.

2. Sympathetic Regulation of Hepatic Glucose Production:

   - Sympathetic innervation of the liver can modulate hepatic glucose production by regulating the activity of key enzymes involved in gluconeogenesis and glycogenolysis.

   - Sympathetic activation may enhance glycogenolysis and gluconeogenesis in the liver, increasing blood glucose levels to meet energy demands during stress or physical exertion.

   - Conversely, sympathetic inhibition may reduce hepatic glucose output, conserving glucose for essential functions and preventing hyperglycemia.

Clinical Implications:

Dysregulation of blood glucose regulation can lead to the development of metabolic disorders such as diabetes mellitus, characterized by aberrant glucose metabolism and impaired insulin action. Understanding the physiological mechanisms underlying blood glucose regulation is essential for elucidating the pathophysiology of diabetes and other metabolic disorders, as well as for developing targeted therapeutic interventions aimed at restoring glucose homeostasis.

10.5 Conclusion:

The physiology of the endocrine pancreas and glucose metabolism is a dynamic and intricately regulated process vital for maintaining metabolic homeostasis in the body. Throughout this chapter, we have explored the complex interplay between insulin, glucagon, and other hormones in modulating blood glucose levels and coordinating metabolic responses to various physiological conditions.

Insulin, synthesized and secreted by pancreatic beta cells, acts as a key regulator of glucose uptake, glycogen synthesis, and protein metabolism in target tissues such as muscle, adipose tissue, and liver. Its actions promote the storage and utilization of glucose, thereby lowering blood glucose levels and providing energy for cellular functions.

Conversely, glucagon, produced by pancreatic alpha cells, counteracts the effects of insulin by stimulating glycogenolysis, gluconeogenesis, and lipolysis, mobilizing glucose and fatty acids from storage sites to maintain blood glucose levels during fasting or stress.

The balance between insulin and glucagon, finely tuned by feedback mechanisms and other hormonal signals, ensures the maintenance of blood glucose levels within a narrow physiological range, essential for cellular function and overall health.

Understanding the physiology of the endocrine pancreas and glucose metabolism is crucial for elucidating the pathophysiology of metabolic disorders such as diabetes mellitus, where dysregulation of insulin secretion or action leads to aberrant glucose homeostasis and associated complications.

Future research in this field holds promise for the development of novel therapeutic interventions aimed at restoring or enhancing pancreatic hormone secretion, improving insulin sensitivity, and optimizing glucose metabolism to mitigate the burden of metabolic diseases on global health.

In conclusion, a comprehensive understanding of the physiology of the endocrine pancreas and glucose metabolism not only advances our knowledge of fundamental biological processes but also offers potential avenues for innovative approaches to disease management and prevention.

Case Studies

Case Study 1: Insulin Deficiency and Diabetes Mellitus

Patient Profile:

- Name: Mary Johnson

- Age: 58 years

- Sex: Female

- Occupation: Retired teacher

- Medical History: Hypertension, obesity

- Family History: Mother had type 2 diabetes

Presentation:

Mary presents with symptoms of increased thirst, frequent urination, and unexplained weight loss over the past few months. She reports feeling extremely tired and experiencing blurred vision. Her diet has been high in carbohydrates, and she leads a sedentary lifestyle.

Physical Examination:

- Vital Signs: BP: 150/95 mmHg, HR: 80 bpm, Temp: 37°C

- General Appearance: Overweight, appears fatigued

- Skin: Dry skin, signs of acanthosis nigricans (dark, velvety skin patches)

- Neurological Exam: Reduced sensation in feet

Laboratory Tests:

- Fasting Blood Glucose: 190 mg/dL

- HbA1c (Glycated Hemoglobin): 8.5%

- Insulin Levels: Low

- C-Peptide Levels: Low

Discussion:

Mary's symptoms, combined with her laboratory results, suggest type 2 diabetes mellitus, characterized by insulin resistance and eventual pancreatic beta-cell dysfunction leading to insulin deficiency.

Questions:

1. Explain the role of insulin in glucose metabolism.

2. Describe the pathophysiology of type 2 diabetes mellitus.

3. What is the significance of measuring HbA1c in diabetic patients?

4. Discuss the potential complications of poorly managed diabetes.

Case Study 2: Hypoglycemia in a Type 1 Diabetic Patient

Patient Profile:

- Name: Tom Smith

- Age: 25 years

- Sex: Male

- Occupation: College student

- Medical History: Type 1 diabetes mellitus (diagnosed at age 12)

- Family History: Father has type 1 diabetes

Presentation:

Tom presents to the emergency department with symptoms of sweating, palpitations, confusion, and dizziness. He reports that he has been adhering to his insulin regimen but missed a meal before his symptoms started.

Physical Examination:

- Vital Signs: BP: 110/70 mmHg, HR: 95 bpm, Temp: 36.7°C

- General Appearance: Appears anxious and confused

- Neurological Exam: Slightly disoriented, but responsive

Laboratory Tests:

- Blood Glucose: 50 mg/dL

- Insulin Levels: High (due to exogenous insulin)

- C-Peptide Levels: Low (indicative of endogenous insulin deficiency)

Discussion:

Tom's symptoms and low blood glucose level indicate hypoglycemia, a common complication in type 1 diabetic patients, particularly when insulin administration is not balanced with carbohydrate intake.

Questions:

1. Explain the physiological mechanisms that prevent hypoglycemia.

2. Describe the symptoms and immediate treatment of hypoglycemia.

3. Discuss the importance of balancing insulin administration with food intake in type 1 diabetes.

4. What are the long-term risks associated with frequent hypoglycemic episodes?

Practice Questions for Self-Assessment

Multiple Choice Questions

1. Which of the following hormones is primarily responsible for lowering blood glucose levels?

    a) Glucagon

    b) Cortisol

    c) Insulin

    d) Epinephrine

2. What is the primary function of glucagon?

    a) Increase blood glucose levels

    b) Decrease blood glucose levels

    c) Stimulate fat storage

    d) Inhibit gluconeogenesis

3. Which of the following is NOT a symptom of diabetes mellitus?

    a) Polyuria

    b) Polydipsia

    c) Polyphagia

    d) Bradycardia

4. What is the primary source of glucose production during fasting?

   a) Glycogenolysis

   b) Lipolysis

   c) Protein synthesis

   d) Ketogenesis

5. Which type of diabetes is characterized by insulin resistance?

   a) Type 1 diabetes

   b) Type 2 diabetes

   c) Gestational diabetes

   d) Maturity-onset diabetes of the young (MODY)

Short Answer Questions

1. Define the role of the endocrine pancreas in glucose metabolism.

2. Explain the difference between type 1 and type 2 diabetes mellitus.

3. Describe the process of glycogenolysis and its importance in glucose homeostasis.

4. Discuss the effects of insulin on lipid metabolism.

5. Explain how exercise influences blood glucose levels in diabetic patients.

True or False Questions

1. Insulin is produced by the alpha cells of the pancreas. (True/False)

2. Glucagon promotes glycogen synthesis in the liver. (True/False)

3. Type 1 diabetes is an autoimmune condition. (True/False)

4. Oral hypoglycemic agents are typically used to manage type 2 diabetes. (True/False)

5. Insulin resistance is a hallmark of type 1 diabetes. (True/False)

Answers

Case Study 1

1. Role of Insulin in Glucose Metabolism:

   - Insulin facilitates the uptake of glucose by cells, particularly muscle and adipose tissues, by binding to insulin receptors and promoting glucose transporter (GLUT4) translocation to the cell membrane. It also inhibits hepatic glucose production and promotes glycogen synthesis, lowering blood glucose levels.

2. Pathophysiology of Type 2 Diabetes Mellitus:

   - Type 2 diabetes is characterized by insulin resistance, where body cells become less responsive to insulin. Over time, the pancreatic beta cells become dysfunctional and fail to produce enough insulin to compensate for the increased demand, leading to hyperglycemia.

3. Significance of Measuring HbA1c:

   - HbA1c reflects the average blood glucose levels over the past 2-3 months, providing a long-term indicator of blood glucose control. It helps assess the effectiveness of diabetes management and the risk of complications.

4. Potential Complications of Poorly Managed Diabetes:

   - Poorly managed diabetes can lead to chronic complications, including cardiovascular disease, neuropathy, nephropathy, retinopathy, and increased risk of infections. Acute complications include diabetic ketoacidosis and hyperosmolar hyperglycemic state.

Case Study 2

1. Physiological Mechanisms Preventing Hypoglycemia:

   - The body prevents hypoglycemia through the actions of counterregulatory hormones such as glucagon, epinephrine, cortisol, and growth hormone, which stimulate hepatic glucose production and inhibit insulin-mediated glucose uptake.

2. Symptoms and Immediate Treatment of Hypoglycemia:

   - Symptoms include sweating, palpitations, tremors, confusion, and dizziness. Immediate treatment involves consuming fast-acting carbohydrates (e.g., glucose tablets, fruit juice) to rapidly increase blood glucose levels.

3. Balancing Insulin Administration with Food Intake:

- In type 1 diabetes, exogenous insulin administration must be carefully balanced with carbohydrate intake to avoid hypoglycemia. This involves adjusting insulin doses based on meal size, carbohydrate content, and physical activity levels.

4. Long-Term Risks of Frequent Hypoglycemic Episodes:

- Frequent hypoglycemia can lead to hypoglycemia unawareness, cognitive impairment, and increased risk of severe hypoglycemic episodes. It can also impact the patient's quality of life and mental health.

Multiple Choice Questions

1. c) Insulin

2. a) Increase blood glucose levels

3. d) Bradycardia

4. a) Glycogenolysis

5. b) Type 2 diabetes

Short Answer Questions

1. Role of Endocrine Pancreas in Glucose Metabolism:

- The endocrine pancreas regulates blood glucose levels through the secretion of insulin and glucagon from the beta and alpha cells of the islets of Langerhans, respectively. Insulin lowers blood glucose by promoting cellular uptake, while glucagon raises blood glucose by stimulating hepatic glucose production.

2. Difference Between Type 1 and Type 2 Diabetes:

- Type 1 diabetes is an autoimmune condition where the immune system attacks and destroys pancreatic beta cells, leading to absolute insulin deficiency. Type 2 diabetes involves insulin resistance and relative insulin deficiency, often associated with obesity and metabolic syndrome.

3. Glycogenolysis Process:

- Glycogenolysis is the breakdown of glycogen to glucose-1-phosphate, which is then converted to glucose-6-phosphate and subsequently to glucose, released into the bloodstream to maintain blood glucose levels during fasting.

4. Effects of Insulin on Lipid Metabolism:

- Insulin promotes lipogenesis (fat synthesis) and inhibits lipolysis (fat breakdown). It stimulates the uptake of fatty acids and glucose by adipocytes, promoting triglyceride storage and reducing circulating free fatty acids.

5. Exercise and Blood Glucose Levels:

- Exercise increases glucose uptake by muscle cells through insulin-independent pathways, reducing blood glucose levels. It also enhances insulin sensitivity, helping to improve blood glucose control in diabetic patients.

True or False Questions

1. False

2. False

3. True

4. True

5. False

Bibliography

1. Campbell, J. E., & Drucker, D. J. (2015). Islet α cells and glucagon--critical regulators of energy homeostasis. Nature Reviews Endocrinology, 11(6), 329-338.

- This review article discusses the critical role of islet α cells and glucagon in energy homeostasis, detailing the mechanisms of glucagon secretion and action.

2. Cherrington, A. D., Moore, M. C., Sindelar, D. K., & Edgerton, D. S. (2007). Insulin action on the liver in vivo. Biochemical Society Transactions, 35(Pt 5), 1171-1174.

- This paper provides insights into the action of insulin on the liver, emphasizing its role in regulating glucose metabolism.

3. Ganong, W. F. (2018). Review of Medical Physiology (26th ed.). McGraw-Hill Education.

- A comprehensive textbook that covers the fundamentals of medical physiology, including detailed chapters on the endocrine pancreas and glucose metabolism.

4. Gerich, J. E. (2010). Role of the kidney in normal glucose homeostasis and in the hyperglycaemia of diabetes mellitus: therapeutic implications. Diabetic Medicine, 27(2), 136-142.

   - This article explores the role of the kidney in glucose homeostasis and its implications for diabetes treatment.

5. Guyton, A. C., & Hall, J. E. (2020). Textbook of Medical Physiology (14th ed.). Elsevier.

   - A widely used physiology textbook that includes detailed sections on the endocrine pancreas, insulin, and glucagon.

6. Magnuson, M. A., & Tokhtaeva, E. (2018). Pancreatic β-cell function and failure in type 2 diabetes. Cold Spring Harbor Perspectives in Medicine, 8(5), a031286.

   - This review focuses on pancreatic β-cell function and the mechanisms leading to β-cell failure in type 2 diabetes.

7. McCulloch, L. J., van de Bunt, M., Braun, M., Frayn, K. N., Clark, A., & Gloyn, A. L. (2011). GLUT2 (SLC2A2) is not the principal glucose sensor in human pancreatic β-cells. Diabetologia, 54(4), 654-662.

   - This research article challenges the traditional view of GLUT2 as the primary glucose sensor in human pancreatic β-cells.

8. Muoio, D. M., & Newgard, C. B. (2008). Mechanisms of disease: molecular and metabolic mechanisms of insulin resistance and β-cell failure in type 2 diabetes. Nature Reviews Molecular Cell Biology, 9(3), 193-205.

   - A detailed review of the molecular and metabolic mechanisms underlying insulin resistance and β-cell failure in type 2 diabetes.

9. Polonsky, K. S. (2012). The past 200 years in diabetes. New England Journal of Medicine, 367(14), 1332-1340.

   - This article provides a historical overview of diabetes research and the progress made in understanding and treating the disease.

10. Rorsman, P., & Ashcroft, F. M. (2018). Pancreatic β-cell electrical activity and insulin secretion: of mice and men. Physiological Reviews, 98(1), 117-214.

    - An in-depth review of the electrical activity of pancreatic β-cells and the mechanisms of insulin secretion, comparing findings from mouse models and human studies.

11. Saltiel, A. R., & Kahn, C. R. (2001). Insulin signalling and the regulation of glucose and lipid metabolism. Nature, 414(6865), 799-806.

- This seminal review discusses the insulin signaling pathways and their roles in regulating glucose and lipid metabolism.

12. Stumvoll, M., Goldstein, B. J., & van Haeften, T. W. (2005). Type 2 diabetes: principles of pathogenesis and therapy. Lancet, 365(9467), 1333-1346.

- A comprehensive review of the pathogenesis and therapeutic approaches for type 2 diabetes.

13. Vaughan, M., & Berger, J. (2017). Pancreatic Hormones and Diabetes Mellitus (8th ed.). Lippincott Williams & Wilkins.

- A textbook focusing specifically on pancreatic hormones and their role in diabetes, providing detailed mechanisms and clinical perspectives.

Chapter 11

Physiology of Parathyroid Glands and Calcium Metabolism

11.1 Anatomy and Histology of Parathyroid Glands: Exploring the Endocrine Regulators of Calcium Homeostasis

The parathyroid glands, often overshadowed by their larger neighbor, the thyroid gland, play a crucial role in maintaining calcium homeostasis in the body. Despite their small size, these endocrine glands exert significant influence over physiological processes through the synthesis and secretion of parathyroid hormone (PTH). This comprehensive exploration delves into the intricate anatomy and histology of the parathyroid glands, shedding light on their structural features, cellular composition, and functional significance in regulating calcium metabolism.

Anatomy of Parathyroid Glands:

The parathyroid glands are typically found in pairs, with each individual possessing four glands, though variations in number and location can occur. Positioned on the posterior surface of the thyroid gland, the parathyroid glands are strategically located to monitor and respond to changes in blood calcium levels. They are often divided into superior and inferior pairs, with the superior glands typically situated near the upper poles of the thyroid gland and the inferior glands near the lower poles. This anatomical arrangement ensures proximity to the thyroid gland's vascular supply, primarily derived from branches of the inferior thyroid artery, facilitating nutrient and oxygen delivery essential for glandular function.

Histology of Parathyroid Glands:

Microscopic examination reveals a specialized cellular composition within the parathyroid glands, reflecting their endocrine function in calcium regulation. The predominant cell type, chief cells, are responsible for synthesizing and secreting PTH, the primary hormone involved in calcium homeostasis. Chief cells exhibit distinctive morphological features, appearing as small, polygonal cells with centrally located nuclei and eosinophilic cytoplasm. This cellular arrangement optimizes the efficiency of PTH synthesis and secretion in response to fluctuations in extracellular calcium levels, ensuring rapid and precise hormonal regulation.

In addition to chief cells, the parathyroid glands contain another cell type known as oxyphil cells. Oxyphil cells are larger and less numerous than chief cells and are characterized by their abundant eosinophilic cytoplasm and centrally located nuclei. Despite their prevalence, the precise function of oxyphil cells remains enigmatic, with hypotheses suggesting a role in calcium metabolism or as a reserve population of chief cells. Their presence underscores the complexity of parathyroid gland histology and hints at potential functional interactions within the glandular microenvironment.

Functional Significance:

The compact organization of chief cells within the parathyroid glands enables swift and coordinated responses to changes in blood calcium levels. Through a feedback mechanism involving calcium-sensing receptors, chief cells detect alterations in extracellular calcium concentrations and adjust PTH secretion accordingly. Elevated calcium levels inhibit PTH secretion, while decreased calcium levels stimulate PTH production and release. This dynamic interplay ensures the maintenance of optimal blood calcium levels essential for neuromuscular function, bone health, and cellular metabolism.

Furthermore, the close anatomical proximity of the parathyroid glands to the thyroid gland facilitates surgical interventions when necessary. Procedures such as parathyroidectomy, commonly performed to treat hyperparathyroidism, benefit from the glands' accessible location and distinct vascular supply. Understanding the functional significance of parathyroid gland anatomy and histology is crucial for diagnosing and managing disorders of calcium metabolism effectively, ensuring optimal patient outcomes and quality of life.

11.2 Parathyroid Hormone (PTH): Synthesis, Secretion, and Actions

Parathyroid hormone (PTH) is a critical regulator of calcium homeostasis, synthesized and secreted by the chief cells of the parathyroid glands. Its secretion is tightly regulated by extracellular calcium levels through a negative feedback mechanism mediated by calcium-sensing receptors on chief cells.

Synthesis and Secretion:

Parathyroid hormone (PTH) synthesis and secretion are intricate processes that begin within the chief cells of the parathyroid glands. These glands, typically four in number, are small endocrine organs located on the posterior surface of the thyroid gland.

1. Synthesis Cascade:

   - The synthesis of PTH initiates with the transcription of the PTH gene, which produces preproparathyroid hormone (preproPTH). This molecule is synthesized in the rough endoplasmic reticulum (RER) of the chief cells.

   - PreproPTH undergoes cleavage to form proparathyroid hormone (proPTH), a precursor molecule.

   - Further processing of proPTH occurs in the Golgi apparatus, where it is enzymatically cleaved to yield the mature PTH molecule, consisting of 84 amino acids.

2. Regulation of Secretion:

   - The secretion of PTH is primarily regulated by extracellular calcium levels sensed by calcium-sensing receptors (CaSRs) located on the surface of chief cells.

   - When extracellular calcium levels decrease (hypocalcemia), CaSRs detect this change and activate intracellular signaling pathways that stimulate PTH secretion.

   - Conversely, elevated extracellular calcium levels (hypercalcemia) inhibit PTH secretion through negative feedback mechanisms mediated by CaSRs.

Actions of PTH:

Parathyroid hormone (PTH) exerts its physiological effects on target organs, primarily bone, kidneys, and intestines, to regulate calcium homeostasis through various mechanisms:

1. Bone:

   - PTH exerts its most significant effect on bone by stimulating osteoclast activity and bone resorption.

   - Osteoclasts are multinucleated cells responsible for breaking down bone matrix, releasing calcium and phosphate into the bloodstream.

   - PTH also inhibits osteoblast activity, indirectly promoting bone resorption and calcium release.

2. Kidneys:

- In the kidneys, PTH enhances renal calcium reabsorption in the distal tubules, reducing urinary calcium excretion and conserving calcium.

- PTH also stimulates the conversion of 25-hydroxyvitamin D (calcidiol) to its active form, calcitriol (1,25-dihydroxyvitamin D3), in the proximal tubules of the kidneys.

- Calcitriol enhances intestinal calcium absorption, further contributing to calcium homeostasis.

3. Intestines:

- PTH indirectly increases intestinal calcium absorption by stimulating the production of calcitriol in the kidneys.

- Calcitriol enhances the expression of calcium-binding proteins in enterocytes, facilitating calcium transport across the intestinal epithelium.

Regulation of PTH Secretion:

In addition to extracellular calcium levels, several factors influence PTH secretion, including phosphate levels, magnesium levels, and calcitriol.

1. Phosphate Levels:

- High phosphate levels in the blood exert a suppressive effect on PTH secretion, reducing its synthesis and release.

- Conversely, low phosphate levels stimulate PTH secretion, promoting calcium mobilization from bone and enhancing renal calcium reabsorption.

2. Magnesium Levels:

- Magnesium deficiency can impair PTH secretion and responsiveness to hypocalcemia, leading to dysregulated calcium homeostasis.

- Adequate magnesium levels are essential for maintaining PTH secretion and sensitivity to extracellular calcium levels.

3. Calcitriol (Active Vitamin D):

   - Calcitriol acts synergistically with PTH to enhance its effects on calcium metabolism.

   - In addition to stimulating intestinal calcium absorption, calcitriol reinforces renal calcium reabsorption and bone resorption, augmenting PTH's actions.

Clinical Relevance:

Disorders of PTH secretion, such as hyperparathyroidism and hypoparathyroidism, can have significant clinical consequences and require careful management.

1. Hyperparathyroidism:

   - Hyperparathyroidism is characterized by excessive secretion of PTH, resulting in hypercalcemia and associated complications.

   - Primary hyperparathyroidism typically occurs due to adenomas or hyperplasia of the parathyroid glands, leading to autonomous PTH secretion.

   - Secondary hyperparathyroidism may develop in response to chronic hypocalcemia or vitamin D deficiency, resulting in compensatory PTH overproduction.

2. Hypoparathyroidism:

   - Hypoparathyroidism arises from deficient PTH secretion, leading to hypocalcemia and neuromuscular irritability.

   - Causes of hypoparathyroidism include surgical removal of the parathyroid glands, autoimmune destruction, or genetic disorders affecting PTH synthesis or secretion.

11.3 Regulation of Calcium and Phosphate Homeostasis Comprehensive Overview

Calcium and phosphate are vital minerals essential for numerous physiological processes, including bone health, muscle contraction, nerve transmission, and enzyme function. The body tightly regulates the levels of these minerals to maintain homeostasis and ensure optimal cellular function. This comprehensive review delves into the intricate mechanisms involved in the regulation of calcium and phosphate homeostasis, highlighting the roles of parathyroid hormone (PTH), calcitonin, vitamin D, and other factors.

Parathyroid Hormone (PTH):

Parathyroid hormone (PTH) is a key regulator of calcium homeostasis, primarily synthesized and secreted by the parathyroid glands. These small endocrine glands, typically four in number, are located on the posterior surface of the thyroid gland. The secretion of PTH is tightly regulated by calcium-sensing receptors on parathyroid chief cells. When blood calcium levels decrease, these receptors detect the change and stimulate PTH secretion.

Once released into the bloodstream, PTH exerts its effects on target organs to increase blood calcium levels through various mechanisms:

- Stimulating osteoclast activity and bone resorption: PTH binds to receptors on osteoblasts, leading to the activation of osteoclasts and subsequent bone resorption. This process releases calcium from the bone matrix into the bloodstream.

- Enhancing renal tubular reabsorption of calcium: PTH increases the reabsorption of calcium in the kidneys, reducing calcium excretion in the urine.

- Stimulating the production of active vitamin D (calcitriol): PTH stimulates the conversion of inactive vitamin D (cholecalciferol) to its active form, calcitriol, in the kidneys. Calcitriol, in turn, enhances intestinal absorption of calcium and phosphate, further increasing blood calcium levels.

PTH secretion is subject to negative feedback regulation, whereby high blood calcium levels inhibit PTH secretion, while low blood calcium levels stimulate its secretion. This feedback loop helps maintain calcium homeostasis within a narrow physiological range.

Calcitonin:

Calcitonin is produced by the parafollicular or C cells of the thyroid gland and acts as a counter-regulatory hormone to PTH. While its role in calcium regulation is less prominent than that of PTH, calcitonin plays a role in reducing blood calcium levels when they are elevated. When blood calcium levels rise, calcitonin secretion is stimulated, inhibiting osteoclast activity and promoting calcium deposition in bones. Additionally, calcitonin enhances renal excretion of calcium, further reducing blood calcium levels.

Despite its regulatory role, calcitonin's contribution to overall calcium homeostasis is relatively minor compared to that of PTH.

Vitamin D (Calcitriol):

Vitamin D is essential for calcium homeostasis and bone health. It exists in several forms, with vitamin D3 (cholecalciferol) being the most biologically active form. Vitamin D can be obtained from dietary sources, supplements, or synthesized in the skin upon exposure to sunlight (UVB radiation). Once synthesized or ingested, vitamin D undergoes hydroxylation in the liver and kidneys to form its active metabolite, calcitriol.

Calcitriol plays a crucial role in calcium and phosphate homeostasis by:

- Enhancing intestinal absorption of calcium and phosphate: Calcitriol stimulates the expression of proteins involved in calcium and phosphate transport across the intestinal epithelium, promoting their absorption into the bloodstream.

- Regulating bone mineralization: Calcitriol helps maintain adequate calcium and phosphate levels for bone formation and mineralization.

- Modulating PTH secretion: Calcitriol suppresses PTH secretion by negative feedback mechanisms when blood calcium levels are sufficient.

Vitamin D deficiency can impair calcium absorption and lead to hypocalcemia, contributing to bone disorders such as rickets in children and osteomalacia in adults.

Other Factors:

In addition to PTH, calcitonin, and vitamin D, several other factors influence calcium and phosphate homeostasis:

- Magnesium: Magnesium is essential for PTH secretion and serves as a cofactor for enzymes involved in vitamin D metabolism. Magnesium deficiency can impair PTH secretion and contribute to hypocalcemia.

- Phosphate: Phosphate levels are regulated by PTH, calcitriol, and fibroblast growth factor 23 (FGF23). PTH increases renal phosphate excretion, while calcitriol enhances intestinal phosphate absorption. FGF23 acts to reduce phosphate reabsorption in the kidneys, helping to maintain phosphate homeostasis.

- Hormones: Estrogen, glucocorticoids, and growth hormone also influence calcium and phosphate metabolism, albeit to varying degrees.

Regulation and Feedback Loops:

The regulation of calcium and phosphate homeostasis involves complex feedback mechanisms to maintain physiological balance. Negative feedback loops play a crucial role in this regulation, ensuring that blood calcium levels remain within a narrow range. When blood calcium levels rise, PTH secretion is inhibited, leading to decreased bone resorption, increased renal calcium excretion, and reduced calcitriol synthesis. Conversely, when blood calcium levels drop, PTH secretion is stimulated, leading to increased bone resorption, enhanced renal calcium reabsorption, and increased calcitriol synthesis.

11.4 Disorders of Parathyroid Glands and Calcium Metabolism

The parathyroid glands are four small endocrine glands located on the posterior surface of the thyroid gland in the neck. Despite their small size, these glands play a critical role in calcium homeostasis through the secretion of parathyroid hormone (PTH). Disorders affecting the parathyroid glands can lead to significant disturbances in calcium and phosphate metabolism, resulting in a range of clinical manifestations. This comprehensive review explores in detail the disorders of parathyroid glands and their impact on calcium metabolism, including primary hyperparathyroidism, secondary hyperparathyroidism, hypoparathyroidism, familial hypocalciuric hypercalcemia (FHH), and pseudohypoparathyroidism.

Primary Hyperparathyroidism

Primary hyperparathyroidism (PHPT) is characterized by excessive secretion of parathyroid hormone (PTH) from one or more of the parathyroid glands. The most common cause of PHPT is a benign tumor (adenoma) in one of the parathyroid glands, although less commonly, hyperplasia of multiple glands or, rarely, parathyroid carcinoma can be the cause.

Pathophysiology

In primary hyperparathyroidism, the overproduction of PTH leads to hypercalcemia and hypophosphatemia. PTH acts on bones, kidneys, and intestines to increase calcium levels in the bloodstream. Increased bone resorption releases calcium into the bloodstream, while renal tubular reabsorption of calcium is enhanced, leading to hypercalcemia.

Clinical Manifestations

The clinical manifestations of primary hyperparathyroidism are often nonspecific and may include:

- Bone pain and fragility fractures due to osteoclastic bone resorption.

- Renal complications such as nephrolithiasis (kidney stones) due to increased urinary calcium excretion.

- Gastrointestinal symptoms like constipation, nausea, and abdominal pain.

- Neuropsychiatric symptoms including fatigue, weakness, and depression.

Diagnosis

Diagnosis of primary hyperparathyroidism involves:

- Measurement of serum calcium levels, which are typically elevated.

- Assessment of PTH levels, which are inappropriately elevated in the setting of hypercalcemia.

- Imaging studies such as neck ultrasound, sestamibi scan, or CT/MRI for localization of adenoma or hyperplasia.

Treatment

The management of primary hyperparathyroidism depends on the severity of symptoms and the presence of complications:

- Surgery (parathyroidectomy) is the definitive treatment for symptomatic primary hyperparathyroidism or when certain criteria for surgery are met (e.g., serum calcium above a certain threshold, reduced bone density).

- Medical management includes hydration, loop diuretics (to promote urinary calcium excretion), and bisphosphonates (for bone protection) in select cases.

Secondary Hyperparathyroidism

Secondary hyperparathyroidism develops as a compensatory response to chronic hypocalcemia and vitamin D deficiency, often due to renal failure or malabsorption.

Pathophysiology

In secondary hyperparathyroidism, decreased calcium levels stimulate the parathyroid glands to produce and secrete more PTH. The goal is to increase serum calcium levels by mobilizing calcium from bones and enhancing renal calcium reabsorption.

Clinical Manifestations

Clinical features of secondary hyperparathyroidism may include:

- Bone abnormalities such as osteitis fibrosa cystica (excessive bone resorption) and osteomalacia (softening of bones).

- Renal osteodystrophy due to disturbances in calcium and phosphate metabolism.

- Symptoms related to underlying renal disease or malabsorption.

Diagnosis

Diagnosis of secondary hyperparathyroidism involves:

- Measurement of serum calcium and phosphate levels, which are typically low.

- Assessment of PTH levels, which are elevated in response to hypocalcemia.

- Evaluation of underlying causes such as renal function tests, vitamin D levels, and imaging studies.

Treatment

The management of secondary hyperparathyroidism aims to address the underlying cause while managing associated complications:

- Correction of vitamin D deficiency and supplementation with active vitamin D analogs.

- Phosphate binders to control hyperphosphatemia.

- Renal replacement therapy (dialysis) in patients with end-stage renal disease.

- Parathyroidectomy may be considered in refractory cases.

Hypoparathyroidism

Hypoparathyroidism results from inadequate secretion of parathyroid hormone (PTH) due to damage or surgical removal of the parathyroid glands.

Pathophysiology

In hypoparathyroidism, the absence or deficiency of PTH leads to hypocalcemia and hyperphosphatemia. Without PTH, renal calcium reabsorption is decreased, leading to increased renal excretion of calcium and phosphate.

Clinical Manifestations

Clinical features of hypoparathyroidism may include:

- Neuromuscular irritability, tetany, muscle cramps, and spasms due to hypocalcemia.

- Paresthesias (tingling sensations), seizures, and psychiatric symptoms in severe cases.

- Chvostek's sign (facial muscle twitching) and Trousseau's sign (carpal spasm) may be elicited on physical examination.

Diagnosis

Diagnosis of hypoparathyroidism involves:

- Measurement of serum calcium and phosphate levels, which are typically low.

- Assessment of PTH levels, which are decreased or undetectable.

- Electrocardiography (ECG) to evaluate for QT interval prolongation.

Treatment

The management of hypoparathyroidism focuses on restoring calcium and phosphate balance:

- Oral calcium supplements and active vitamin D analogs to raise and maintain serum calcium levels.

- Long-term monitoring and adjustment of medications to prevent complications such as hypercalciuria and nephrocalcinosis.

Familial Hypocalciuric Hypercalcemia (FHH)

Familial hypocalciuric hypercalcemia (FHH) is an autosomal dominant disorder characterized by mild hypercalcemia and hypocalciuria due to mutations in the calcium-sensing receptor (CaSR).

Pathophysiology

In FHH, mutations in the CaSR result in reduced sensitivity to extracellular calcium levels, leading to inappropriate PTH secretion despite normal or elevated serum calcium levels.

Clinical Manifestations

FHH is typically asymptomatic or associated with mild nonspecific symptoms, such as fatigue or constipation.

Diagnosis

Diagnosis of FHH involves:

- Measurement of serum calcium and PTH levels, which are typically mildly elevated.

- Assessment of urinary calcium excretion, which is low despite hypercalcemia.

- Genetic testing to identify mutations in the CaSR gene.

Treatment

Management of FHH is generally conservative, focusing on monitoring and surveillance for potential complications such as hypercalcemia-related disorders.

Pseudohypoparathyroidism

Pseudohypoparathyroidism refers to a group of rare genetic disorders characterized by target organ resistance to the actions of PTH despite normal or elevated circulating levels of the hormone.

Pathophysiology

In pseudohypoparathyroidism, mutations in the PTH receptor or downstream signaling pathways impair the cellular response to PTH, leading to hypocalcemia and hyperphosphatemia.

Clinical Manifestations

Clinical features of pseudohypoparathyroidism may resemble those of hypoparathyroidism, including neuromuscular irritability, tetany, and seizures.

Diagnosis

Diagnosis of pseudohypoparathyroidism involves:

- Measurement of serum calcium and phosphate levels, which may be low or normal.

- Assessment of PTH levels, which are typically elevated despite hypocalcemia.

- Evaluation for features of Albright hereditary osteodystrophy (AHO), such as short stature and brachydactyly.

Treatment

The management of pseudohypoparathyroidism is similar to that of hypoparathyroidism and involves supplementation with oral calcium and active vitamin D analogs to maintain serum calcium levels within the normal range.

11.4 Conclusion:

The parathyroid glands and parathyroid hormone play critical roles in the regulation of calcium and phosphate homeostasis. Through their actions on bone, kidney, and intestine, PTH ensures the maintenance of optimal blood calcium levels essential for neuromuscular function, bone health, and overall physiological well-being. Understanding the physiology of parathyroid glands and calcium metabolism is essential for diagnosing and managing disorders of calcium homeostasis effectively.

Case Studies

Case Study 1: Hyperparathyroidism and Hypercalcemia

Patient Profile:

- Name: Mary Johnson

- Age: 55 years

- Sex: Female

- Occupation: Retired Teacher

- Medical History: Osteoporosis, kidney stones

- Family History: Mother had osteoporosis

Presentation:

Mary presents to her primary care physician with complaints of bone pain, frequent urination, and muscle weakness. She also mentions that she has been experiencing increased thirst and digestive issues, including constipation.

Physical Examination:

- Vital Signs: BP: 130/80 mmHg, HR: 72 bpm, Temp: 37°C

- General Appearance: Normal weight, appears slightly dehydrated

- Musculoskeletal: Tenderness in bones

- Neurological: Muscle weakness, decreased reflexes

Laboratory Tests:

- Serum Calcium: Elevated

- Parathyroid Hormone (PTH): Elevated

- Serum Phosphate: Low

- 25-hydroxy Vitamin D: Normal

Imaging:

- Bone Density Scan: Reduced bone density indicative of osteoporosis

- Neck Ultrasound: Enlarged parathyroid gland

Discussion:

Mary's elevated serum calcium and PTH levels, along with her symptoms, suggest primary hyperparathyroidism. This condition is characterized by excessive secretion of PTH, leading to hypercalcemia and subsequent complications such as osteoporosis and kidney stones.

Questions:

1. Explain the role of PTH in calcium homeostasis.

2. What are the effects of elevated PTH on bones, kidneys, and the gastrointestinal system?

3. Discuss the feedback mechanism involved in regulating PTH secretion.

4. How does primary hyperparathyroidism lead to hypercalcemia?

Case Study 2: Hypoparathyroidism and Hypocalcemia

Patient Profile:

- Name: James Smith

- Age: 40 years

- Sex: Male

- Occupation: Construction Worker

- Medical History: Thyroid surgery for thyroid cancer

- Family History: No significant medical history

Presentation:

James presents to the emergency department with tingling and numbness in his hands and feet, muscle cramps, and a sensation of difficulty breathing. He also reports having occasional seizures over the past few days.

Physical Examination:

- Vital Signs: BP: 120/75 mmHg, HR: 80 bpm, Temp: 36.5°C

- Neurological: Positive Chvostek's sign, positive Trousseau's sign

- Musculoskeletal: Muscle cramps and spasms

- Respiratory: Mild respiratory distress

Laboratory Tests:

- Serum Calcium: Low

- Parathyroid Hormone (PTH): Low

- Scrum Phosphate: Elevated

- Magnesium: Normal

Imaging:

- Neck Ultrasound: Post-surgical changes, no residual thyroid or parathyroid tissue observed

Discussion:

James' symptoms and lab results indicate hypoparathyroidism, likely a result of inadvertent removal or damage to the parathyroid glands during thyroid surgery. The condition leads to hypocalcemia, causing neuromuscular irritability and other related symptoms.

Questions:

1. Describe the role of PTH in maintaining serum calcium levels.

2. What are the clinical manifestations of hypocalcemia?

3. Explain how the feedback mechanism for PTH secretion works.

4. How does hypoparathyroidism lead to hypocalcemia?

Practice Questions for Self-Assessment

Multiple Choice Questions

1. Which of the following is a direct action of parathyroid hormone (PTH)?

　a) Decreasing calcium reabsorption in the kidneys

b) Increasing phosphate reabsorption in the kidneys

c) Stimulating osteoclast activity in bones

d) Decreasing vitamin D activation in the kidneys

2. Which condition is characterized by low levels of PTH?

a) Hyperthyroidism

b) Hyperparathyroidism

c) Hypoparathyroidism

d) Cushing's syndrome

3. Which vitamin is crucial for the proper function of PTH?

a) Vitamin A

b) Vitamin B12

c) Vitamin D

d) Vitamin K

4. The primary function of PTH in bone is to:

a) Promote bone formation

b) Stimulate osteoclast activity

c) Inhibit osteoblast activity

d) Increase calcium deposition in bones

5. Which of the following is a symptom of hypercalcemia?

a) Muscle spasms

b) Bone pain

c) Dry skin

d) Increased appetite

Short Answer Questions

1. Define the primary function of the parathyroid glands.

2. Explain the role of calcium in the human body.

3. Describe the process of calcium regulation by PTH and vitamin D.

4. Discuss the potential complications of untreated hyperparathyroidism.

5. Explain the symptoms and treatment options for hypocalcemia.

True or False Questions

1. PTH increases calcium absorption in the intestines. (True/False)

2. Hyperparathyroidism can lead to kidney stones. (True/False)

3. Hypocalcemia is commonly associated with high serum phosphate levels. (True/False)

4. Vitamin D deficiency can exacerbate hypocalcemia. (True/False)

5. PTH secretion is directly stimulated by high serum calcium levels. (True/False)

Answers

Case Study 1

1. Feedback Mechanism in PTH Regulation:

   - In response to low blood calcium levels, the parathyroid glands secrete PTH, which increases calcium release from bones, reabsorption in kidneys, and absorption in the intestines. Elevated blood calcium levels inhibit PTH release through a negative feedback loop, maintaining calcium homeostasis.

2. Role of PTH:

   - PTH regulates calcium and phosphate metabolism by increasing blood calcium levels and decreasing blood phosphate levels. It acts on bones, kidneys, and the intestine to achieve these effects.

3. Physiological Effects of Calcium:

   - Calcium is vital for muscle contraction, blood clotting, nerve transmission, and bone strength. It also acts as a secondary messenger in various cellular processes.

4. Vitamin D and Calcium Regulation:

   - Vitamin D enhances calcium absorption in the intestines and works with PTH to regulate blood calcium levels. It is converted to its active form, calcitriol, in the kidneys under PTH influence.

Case Study 2

1. Role of Calcitonin in Calcium Homeostasis:

   - Calcitonin, produced by the thyroid gland, lowers blood calcium levels by inhibiting bone resorption and enhancing calcium excretion by the kidneys. It acts antagonistically to PTH.

2. Mechanism of Action of Calcitonin:

- Calcitonin binds to receptors on osteoclasts, inhibiting their activity and reducing bone resorption. It also promotes calcium excretion in the kidneys, lowering blood calcium levels.

3. Regulation of Blood Calcium Levels:

- Blood calcium levels are regulated by the interplay between PTH, calcitonin, and vitamin D. PTH and vitamin D increase calcium levels, while calcitonin decreases them.

4. Impact of Prolonged Hypercalcemia:

- Prolonged hypercalcemia can lead to kidney stones, bone pain, and neurological issues such as confusion and lethargy. It can also cause arrhythmias and calcification of soft tissues.

Multiple Choice Questions

1. c) Regulate calcium levels in the blood

2. a) Parathyroid hormone (PTH)

3. b) Calcitonin

4. d) Bone, kidney, intestine

5. c) Calcitriol

Short Answer Questions

1. Parathyroid Hormone (PTH):

- PTH increases blood calcium levels by stimulating bone resorption, increasing renal reabsorption of calcium, and enhancing intestinal absorption of calcium through activation of vitamin D.

2. Role of Vitamin D:

- Vitamin D is essential for calcium absorption in the intestines. It is converted to its active form, calcitriol, in the kidneys under the influence of PTH, and it helps maintain appropriate calcium and phosphate levels in the blood.

3. Calcitonin and Calcium Homeostasis:

  - Calcitonin, produced by the thyroid gland, lowers blood calcium levels by inhibiting bone resorption and increasing calcium excretion by the kidneys, counteracting the effects of PTH.

4. Calcium Regulation Mechanisms:

  - Blood calcium levels are regulated through the actions of PTH, calcitonin, and vitamin D. PTH and vitamin D increase calcium levels, while calcitonin decreases them, maintaining homeostasis.

5. Impact of Hyperparathyroidism:

  - Hyperparathyroidism leads to excessive PTH secretion, causing hypercalcemia, weakened bones, kidney stones, and neuropsychiatric disturbances due to elevated blood calcium levels.

True or False Questions

1. True

2. True

3. False

4. True

5. True

Bibliography

1. Bilezikian, J. P., & Khan, A. (Eds.). (2019). Principles of Bone Biology (4th ed.). Academic Press.

   - This comprehensive textbook covers the physiology of parathyroid glands, calcium metabolism, and disorders related to bone and mineral metabolism.

2. Bringhurst, F. R., Demay, M. B., & Kronenberg, H. M. (Eds.). (2016). Williams Textbook of Endocrinology (13th ed.). Elsevier.

   - Provides detailed insights into parathyroid hormone physiology, calcium homeostasis, and clinical disorders involving parathyroid glands.

3. Kovacs, C. S., & Kronenberg, H. M. (2019). Disorders of Bone and Mineral Metabolism. In J. L. Jameson, J. O. L. De Groot, D. L. de Kretser, L. J. Grossman, R. P. Auchus, & G. D. Chrousos (Eds.), Endocrinology: Adult and Pediatric (8th ed., pp. 1075-1113). Elsevier.

   - A comprehensive chapter that discusses parathyroid hormone physiology, regulation of calcium and phosphate metabolism, and clinical disorders.

4. Silverberg, S. J., & Bilezikian, J. P. (2019). Primary hyperparathyroidism. In J. P. Bilezikian, C. T. Peacock, & A. P. Rosen (Eds.), The Parathyroids (3rd ed., pp. 423-452). Elsevier.

   - Focuses on primary hyperparathyroidism, including epidemiology, pathophysiology, diagnosis, and management.

5. Walker, M. D., & Silverberg, S. J. (2020). Bone disease in primary hyperparathyroidism. Journal of Bone and Mineral Research, 35(12), 2229-2240. https://doi.org/10.1002/jbmr.4076

   - Discusses bone disease associated with primary hyperparathyroidism, with insights into pathogenesis and clinical implications.

Glossary of Key Terms

A

Adenohypophysis (Anterior Pituitary): Front portion of the pituitary gland; secretes GH, PRL, ACTH, TSH, LH, and FSH.

Adrenal Cortex: Outer layer of the adrenal glands; produces cortisol, aldosterone, and androgens.

Adrenal Medulla: Inner part of adrenal glands; produces adrenaline and noradrenaline.

Adrenocorticotropic Hormone (ACTH): Hormone from the anterior pituitary that stimulates the adrenal cortex.

Aldosterone: Mineralocorticoid from the adrenal cortex; regulates sodium, potassium, and blood pressure.

Androgens: Steroid hormones from the adrenal cortex and gonads; contribute to male traits and reproductive activity.

Autocrine Signaling: Cell signaling where a cell targets itself.

B

Basal Metabolic Rate (BMR): Rate of energy expenditure by an organism at rest.

Binding Protein: Proteins that transport hormones in the blood, regulating availability.

C

Catecholamines: Hormones (adrenaline, noradrenaline) from the adrenal medulla; involved in 'fight or flight' response.

Cortisol: Glucocorticoid from the adrenal cortex; regulates metabolism and stress response.

Cyclic AMP (cAMP): Secondary messenger in signal transduction.

Cytokines: Small proteins affecting cell communication and interaction.

D

Diabetes Mellitus: Diseases causing high blood glucose due to insulin issues.

Downregulation: Decrease in hormone receptor numbers/sensitivity due to high hormone levels.

E

Endocrine Glands: Glands secreting hormones into the bloodstream (e.g., pituitary, thyroid, adrenal).

Endocrinology: Study of the endocrine glands and hormones.

Epinephrine (Adrenaline): Hormone from adrenal medulla; increases heart rate and blood pressure.

Estrogens: Steroid hormones promoting female traits and reproductive function.

Exocrine Glands: Glands secreting substances through ducts (e.g., sweat, salivary glands).

F

Feedback Mechanism: Process regulating physiological functions via feedback loops, can be negative or positive.

Follicle-Stimulating Hormone (FSH): Anterior pituitary hormone; promotes formation of ova or sperm.

G

Glucagon: Hormone from pancreatic alpha cells; raises blood glucose levels.

Glucocorticoids: Steroid hormones from the adrenal cortex; affect glucose metabolism and immune response.

Gonadotropins: Hormones (LH, FSH) stimulating gonads.

Growth Hormone (GH): Anterior pituitary hormone; stimulates growth and cell reproduction.

H

Homeostasis: Maintenance of stable internal conditions.

Hormones: Chemical messengers produced by endocrine glands; regulate physiology and behavior.

Hypoglycemia: Low blood glucose levels.

Hypothalamic-Pituitary-Adrenal (HPA) Axis: Interaction between hypothalamus, pituitary gland, and adrenal glands; regulates stress response, digestion, immune system, etc.

Hypothalamus: Brain region controlling many body functions; releases hormones influencing pituitary gland.

I

Insulin: Hormone from pancreatic beta cells; lowers blood glucose levels.

Insulin-like Growth Factors (IGFs): Proteins similar to insulin; play a role in growth and development.

Islets of Langerhans: Pancreatic cell clusters secreting insulin and glucagon.

J

Juxtacrine Signaling: Cell signaling via direct contact.

K

Kallikrein-Kinin System: Blood proteins involved in inflammation, blood pressure control, coagulation, and pain.

L

Leptin: Hormone from fat cells; regulates energy balance by inhibiting hunger.

Luteinizing Hormone (LH): Anterior pituitary hormone; triggers ovulation, stimulates sex hormone production.

M

Melatonin: Pineal gland hormone; regulates sleep-wake cycles.

Metabolism: Chemical processes within a living organism to maintain life, including anabolism and catabolism.

Mineralocorticoids: Corticosteroids influencing salt and water balance (e.g., aldosterone).

N

Neuroendocrine Cells: Cells releasing hormones in response to neuronal input.

Neurohypophysis (Posterior Pituitary): Back portion of the pituitary gland; stores/releases oxytocin and vasopressin.

Noradrenaline (Norepinephrine): Catecholamine from adrenal medulla; functions as neurotransmitter and hormone.

O

Oxytocin: Hormone from hypothalamus; stimulates uterine contractions, milk ejection.

P

Paracrine Signaling: Cell signaling where the target cell is nearby the signal-releasing cell.

Parathyroid Glands: Small glands behind the thyroid; produce PTH.

Parathyroid Hormone (PTH): Hormone regulating blood calcium levels.

Pineal Gland: Small brain gland; produces melatonin.

Pituitary Gland: Gland at brain base; produces hormones regulating growth, metabolism, and reproduction.

Prolactin (PRL): Anterior pituitary hormone; stimulates milk production.

R

Radioimmunoassay (RIA): Technique to measure hormone levels using antibodies.

Receptors: Proteins on or in cells that bind hormones, triggering responses.

Renin-Angiotensin-Aldosterone System (RAAS): Hormone system regulating blood pressure and fluid balance.

S

Second Messenger: Molecules relaying signals from receptors to target molecules.

Steroid Hormones: Hormones derived from cholesterol (e.g., sex hormones, adrenal cortex hormones).

Somatostatin: Hormone inhibiting GH and insulin release.

T

Target Cells: Cells with specific receptors for a hormone.

Testosterone: Male sex hormone from testes; regulates fertility, muscle mass, fat distribution, and RBC production.

Thyroid Gland: Neck gland producing hormones regulating metabolism, growth, and development.

Thyroid Hormones: Hormones (T3, T4) from the thyroid; regulate metabolism.

Thyroid-Stimulating Hormone (TSH): Anterior pituitary hormone; stimulates thyroid hormone production.

U

Upregulation: Increase in hormone receptor numbers/sensitivity due to low hormone levels.

V

Vasopressin (Antidiuretic Hormone, ADH): Hormone from hypothalamus; regulates water balance.

W

Water-Soluble Hormones: Hormones soluble in water (e.g., peptide hormones, catecholamines).

White Adipose Tissue: Fat tissue storing energy and producing hormones like leptin.

X

Xenobiotics: Chemical substances foreign to the biological system.

Y

Yohimbine: Alkaloid with stimulant and aphrodisiac properties; blocks alpha-2 adrenergic receptors.

Z

Zona Glomerulosa: Outer adrenal cortex zone; produces aldosterone.

Zona Fasciculata: Middle adrenal cortex zone; produces glucocorticoids like cortisol.

Zona Reticularis: Inner adrenal cortex zone; produces androgens.

Books in the same series

UNDERSTANDING NEURO-PHYSIOLOGY *by Mark Aquino & others*

UNDERSTANDING THE PHYSIOLOGY OF THE CARDIOVASCULAR SYSTEM *by Weber Justin & others*

UNDERSTANDING WORK PHYSIOLOGY *by Elijah Austin & others*

UNDERSTANDING THE PHYSIOLOGY OF THE RESPIRATORY SYSTEM *by Mark Aquino & others*

UNDERSTANDING THE PHYSIOLOGY OF THE RENAL SYSTEM *by Mark Aquino & others*

UNDERSTANDING THE PHYSIOLOGY OF THE ENDOCRINE SYSTEM *by Mark Aquino & others*

Books From The Same Publishers

WEALTH BEYOND MEASURE: Unveiling Biblical Secrets to Prosperity *by Isaiah Opulence*

MASTERING PRODUCTIVITY: How to Use the Eisenhower Matrix for Prioritizing Tasks *by Elijah Yussuf*

MASTERING PRODUCTIVITY: Understanding The "Kaizen"Principles For Continuous Improvement And Optimization *by ELIJAH YUSSUF*

PROCRASTINATORS GUIDE TO PROGRESS: Beating procrastination *by Elijah Yussuf*

THE FORGOTTEN CHILD REMEMBERED: An Autobiography of IFEYORI IHIMODU, FILRM @70 *by Ifeyori Ihimodu*

THE ART OF HYPER-REALISTIC CAKE DESIGN *by Dhebbie Sweet*

MASTERING PRODUCTIVITY: How to the Pomodoro Technique For Time Management *by Elijah Yussuf*

MASTERING THE ART AND CRAFT OF DRIVING: A comprehensive practical guide to driving an Automatic and Manual transmission *by Paul Lucas*

THE MAGICAL BEGINNINGS: Tales Of Whimsy And Wonder *by Qetsy*

FAR FROM HOME: Dreams Beyond Borders *by Qetsy*

CRAFTING WINNING BUSINESS PROPOSALS: A Comprehensive Guide to Success *by* Elight *Yolan.*

12 DAYS OF CHRISTMAS: The Johnson's Family Christmas Tale *by Elijah Yussuf and Sammiel Dickson.*

CRIMSON CAROL: A Candy Cane Thriller *by Qetsy*

ANOINTED WORDS: Inspiring Devotions for Daily Living *by Isaiah Opulence*

Printed in Great Britain
by Amazon

f91d6e4b-279e-4565-8cac-f147ad05c0a2R01